SAW PALMETTO WORKS!

- "Saw palmetto is unbelievable. I get very consistent results. Older men say their frequency at night drops from 3 or 4 to one."

  —Michael Janson, M.D., President of the American College for the Advancement of Medicine

- "My top choice for treating BPH (benign prostate hyperplasia) is saw palmetto. . . . The longest I've had a person on saw palmetto is four years and there's been no side effects reported."

  —Donald Brown, N.D., author of *Herbal Prescriptions for Better Health*

- "I've had a very good response to saw palmetto. Most of the men reported a decrease in symptoms."

  —Cherry Briskey, N.D., clinical faculty president at South West Naturopathic Medical Center in Tempe, Arizona

- "I use saw palmetto as my first choice, in a dose of 160 mg twice a day. If there's no improvement, I either change to a tea form of saw palmetto or the tincture."

  —Lise Alschuler, N.D., Chair of the Botanical Medicine Department at Bastyr University in Seattle, Washington

SAW PALMETTO

NATURE'S PROSTATE HEALER

Ray Sahelian, M.D.

Kensington Books
Kensington Publishing Corp.
http://www.kensingtonbooks.com

KENSINGTON BOOKS are published by

Kensington Publishing Corp.
850 Third Avenue
New York, NY 10022

ISBN 1-57566-300-7

First Kensington Printing: April, 1998
10 9 8 7 6 5 4 3 2 1

Printed in the United States of America

ACKNOWLEDGMENTS

Researchers

James Duke, formally with the United States Department of Agriculture, has been an herbalist for many years, and is the author of *The Green Pharmacy* (Rodale Press, 1997).

Jerry McLaughlin, Ph.D., is Professor of Pharmacognosy, Department of Medicinal Chemistry and Molecular Pharmacology, School of Pharmacy and Pharmacal Sciences, at Purdue University in West Lafayette, Indiana. He has discovered substances within saw palmetto extract, called monolaurin and monomyristin, that have anti-tumor potential.

J. Jeffrey Mullahey, Ph.D., is Associate Professor at the Wildlife Ecology and Conservation at the University of Florida in Immokalee, Florida. He has extensive experience in the growth and harvesting of SP in Florida, and conducts various field studies.

Physicians

Lise Alschuler, N.D., is Chair of the Botanical Medicine Department at Bastyr University in Seattle, Washington. She regularly uses botanical medicines in her clinical practice.

Stan Bazilian, M.D., is a physician in Philadelphia, Pennsylvania.

James Balch, M.D., is a urologist in Trophy Club, Texas. He is also the co-author of *Prescriptions for Natural Healing.*

Marie Bochniak, D.C., is Assistant Clinical Professor at Los Angeles College of Chiropractic.

Donald Brown, N.D., is the author of *Herbal Prescrip-*

tions for Better Health, (Prima, 1996), and President of Natural Product Research Consultants in Seattle, Washington.

Skye Lininger, D.C., is a chiropractic physician in Portland, Oregon.

Bob Martin, D.C., is a chiropractic physician and radio show host on KFYI-AM 910 in Phoenix, Arizona.

Rob McCaleb is President and Founder of Herb Research Foundation in Boulder, Colorado.

Jan McBarron, M.D., is board certified in Preventive Medicine and practices in Columbus, Georgia.

Ascanio Polimeni, M.D., has a private practice in Milan and Rome, Italy.

Richard Podell, M.D., is Director of The Podell Center for Medical Treatment, Prevention, and Natural Healing in New Providence, New Jersey, and Clinical Professor, Department of Family Medicine at UMDMJ-Robert Wood Johnson Medical School in New Brunswick, New Jersey.

Contents

Even My Dad Takes It

My dad is the world's worst patient—a doctor's nightmare. He never follows a physician's advice and never takes any pills he is prescribed. He refuses to take simple vitamins and I've never even seen him medicate with an aspirin for a headache. "My body can heal itself. Why should I take a pill?" is his usual argument. At age 71, he is in relatively good health except for having prostate enlargement and atrial fibrillation (an irregular heartbeat). His doctor prescribed digitalis to return the heartbeat back to normal rhythm. Every time he goes for an appointment, his M.D. checks his pulse and finds the heartbeat to be irregular.

"Are you sure you're taking your medicine?"

"Of course," my dad asserts. "Well, actually, I take it for a few days and feel better so I stop it."

"How can you do that? You're supposed to be on it all the time!"

"Okay, I'll go back on it. I promise."

Fat chance. His bottle of digitalis prescribed over three months ago is still practically full.

My parents live about an hour away from me and normally visit once a month. In March of 1997, as my dad was walking through the kitchen, he saw a bottle of saw palmetto on the counter.

"My neighbor told me about this," he said. "It's supposed to shrink the prostate gland. You're only 39. You're not having prostate problems at your age, are you?"

I had bought a bottle of saw palmetto from a local vitamin store because some of the research I had come across indicated that extracts of this plant were beneficial in reducing the size of the prostate gland. I had also read many articles in magazines discussing the benefits of this plant extract, how much to take, and the proposed mechanism for its actions. Some of this information seemed incomplete or conflicting. I wanted to find out for myself everything there was to know about its medical uses. I've come to a point in my medical career where I'm reluctant to accept any secondhand information. In order to really know a topic, I personally need to read all the basic research papers, treat patients with it, interview other doctors using the supplement, interview top researchers who are experimenting with it, and survey users. A full, comprehensive evaluation of this information would thus satisfy my skeptic and inquiring mind.

In addition, my policy has always been to take a supplement myself for a while before writing about it. I have done so with melatonin, DHEA, creatine, pregnenolone, and glucosamine. There are positive and negative effects regarding the use of supplements that are often not mentioned in the medical literature. Sometimes a great way to find out is experimenting on oneself. A person can gain enormous insights by temporarily taking these supplements. But finding potential side effects wasn't the only reason I was using this plant extract.

"Saw palmetto has been claimed to have an effect

on testosterone and other hormones and I want to see if taking it will have any influence on my hair and skin," I said.

He didn't seem to have heard my reply.

"Does it really work? You know I've been waking up a few times a night to go to the bathroom lately. My doctor recommended I take some pills but I wasn't interested."

"I'm still in the process of fully evaluating the research," I stated. "So far, it seems to be very promising."

That next day, at breakfast, I reached over to my kitchen counter were I keep all my supplements. I usually have about a dozen or so different bottles of multivitamins, antioxidants, zinc lozenges, melatonin, pregnenolone, creatine, and others on the counter. For the past month I had been taking a capsule of saw palmetto twice a day. One by one I went through all the bottles, but the saw palmetto wasn't there. I looked everywhere in the kitchen, and even searched the living room thinking that perhaps my dad had left it on the coffee table. He had seemed quite intrigued by this supplement and had been reading everything written on the label. The bottle was nowhere to be found. I picked up the phone and called my parents. My mom answered.

"Hi mom. Listen, dad was playing with my saw palmetto bottle yesterday. By any chance, do you know where he put it? I searched all over and can't find it."

"He put it in his coat pocket and took it home with him," she said.

"You're kidding. Why didn't he just go to the store and buy his own?"

"Well, it was late when we left your place and all the stores would have been closed. He was very eager to get started on it. He didn't want to wait till the next day to go to the store. He took two capsules last night.''

''That's surprising. He normally never takes any pills.''

''I was surprised, too. But I guess waking up a few times at night to go to the bathroom is wearing him down. He's willing to try almost anything.''

Two weeks later my dad called.

''I think it's working,'' he exclaimed. ''My frequency is less. I'm not waking up as many times to go to the bathroom. My neighbor was right after all.''

I gave a call to Edmund, my dad's 68-year-old neighbor. He seemed extremely pleased with his results.

''I've had an enlarged prostate for many years,'' he told me. ''For the past few months I've been going to the bathroom six times a night. I started saw palmetto 3 months ago. Now I only get up once or twice. I feel fantastic.''

''How long did it take for you to notice the effects?'' I asked.

''It took about a month. My dose was 160 mg twice a day.''

''Have you had any side effects?''

''None so far.''

''How does your doctor feel about you taking it?''

''I belong to a managed care program. Both my private doctor and my urologist know I'm taking it. They're not encouraging me to take it, nor are they discouraging me. I had a PSA (prostatic surface antigen test) done a year ago and it was 6.8. A month after taking saw palmetto, I had the test repeated and the result was 4.5. My doctors are supervising me while I'm on this supplement.

''A retired dentist friend of mine had a TURP

(transurethral resection of the prostate) two years ago for an enlarged prostate. He did well for a while but his problems recurred. He didn't want to have the surgery again. I told him about saw palmetto. He loves it.''

A few months later, my dad, the world's worst pill taker, is still on saw palmetto. So is his neighbor Edmund, and so are countless others who have discovered the benefits of this plant extract.

But what really is saw palmetto? Is it effective, or are most of these older men experiencing a mass illusion? Can saw palmetto be combined with other herbs or drugs to provide relief to anyone suffering from BPH? Is it safe for long-term use? And how does it actually work?

CHAPTER 1

A Brief History of the Berry

Saw palmetto is a dwarf palm tree native to North America and mostly found in Southeastern states such as Florida, Georgia, Louisiana, Mississippi, and South Carolina (Shimada, 1997). It has large leaves that can be up to two feet long, and also has reddish- or brownish-black berries. The Latin name for saw palmetto is *Serenoa repens*.

The medicinal value of saw palmetto has been described in the medical literature since the 1800s. Back in 1898, at least one author reported that tinctures of the fruits and crushed seeds were being used for relief of prostate gland enlargement and possible aphrodisiac qualities (Tanner). It's been reported that American Indian tribes, such as the Seminoles, were quite familiar with saw palmetto and they used the crushed berries in the therapy of certain genito-urinary conditions. Women were also given the berries for certain gynecological problems, including painful periods.

Saw palmetto was a problem to the Europeans who settled in Florida and other Southeastern states (Tanner). Since this plant was resistant to fire, the settlers had a great deal of difficulty in establishing crop fields and pastures. Farmers had to physically

remove each plant. Eventually various types of
mechanical equipment were devised to eradicate the
plant. This was unfortunate for the local wildlife.
Many animals consume the berries and some birds
prefer the plant for nesting and protective cover.
Bears may gorge themselves on saw palmetto fruits.
A road-killed adult female bear in the Ocala National
Forest in Florida was found to have over 30 pounds
of palmetto fruit in her stomach (Tanner).

Commercialization of saw palmetto began in the
1960s when its benefits began being scientifically
explored.

Vive La France

In the 1960s, French researchers, who were familiar with some of the folklore regarding saw palmetto,
started evaluating the chemical constituents of the
berries in order to determine whether any of its his-
torical uses had merit. These researchers eventually
isolated fatty extracts from the berry and formulated
it as a trademarked product called Permixon, which
was released in 1981 (Champault, 1984). The Pierre
Fabré Medicaments company holds this trademark.
Other trademark names include Sereprostat (in
Spain), Prostagutt (by German company Schwabe),
Capistan, Strogen Forte, and Libeprosta (Ravenna,
1996).

Starting in the late 1970s, various research projects
were funded or organized by Pierre Fabré to evaluate
the role of saw palmetto extract (hereafter referred
to as SP) in the therapy of prostate enlargement. Of
course, the trademarked version of SP extract was
used in these studies. After a few successful trials,
Permixon was gradually incorporated into the ther-

apy of prostate symptoms in Europe. It is widely prescribed in many countries, especially France and Germany. The benefits of SP gradually became known in the US and many physicians practicing nutritional or herbal medicine started prescribing SP for their patients with prostate enlargement. Little by little, some of the mainstream media published articles regarding the therapeutic potential of this herb. However, the popularity of a pharmaceutical medicine, Proscar, completely overshadowed SP.

Dozens of American vitamin companies currently sell a non-trademarked version of SP. Many use the actual name of saw palmetto on their bottle while others have made up a specific product name. Most of these companies include 160 mg in their capsule or tablet while others have dosages ranging from 80 mg to 320 mg. Most of the pills are 160 mg because that is the dosage found in the trademarked product Permixon. Many of the studies using SP were done, funded, or sponsored by Pierre Fabré Medicaments, using Permixon. It has not been conclusively proven that 160 mg is the only correct dosage. It's quite possible that a range of dosages could be just as effective, or possibly even more effective.

In 1995, the economic value of SP fruit made the news when the price for the raw fruit exceeded $3 a pound (Tanner, 1997). Previously, SP had been regarded as a pest by many landowners, but the current demand from pharmaceutical and vitamin companies is bound to increase.

CHAPTER 2

The Ps and Qs of Saw Palmetto

What's In SP?

There are a variety of compounds within the SP berry (Fitzpatrick, 1995). As a rule they are divided into four major categories:

1. Free fatty acids. A number of fatty acids are present in SP. The ones in highest concentration include oleic acid, lauric acid, myristic acid and palmitic acid.
2. Phytosterols (plant sterols). These plant sterols (*phyto* means plant) have a chemical structure similar to cholesterol. The most commonly found phytosterols in SP are beta-sitosterol, campesterol, stigmasterol and cycloartenol (Plosker, 1996).
3. Free fatty alcohols. These are usually made up of fatty acids joined to an alcohol molecule.
4. Monoglycerides. These are single fatty acids attached to a three-carbon glycerol molecule (Shimada, 1997).

All of these compounds are fat-soluble. There are several methods for extracting them from the berry.

The most common methods are the use of hexane solvent, carbon dioxide, and ethanol.

According to Dr. Jerry McLaughlin, Professor of Pharmacognosy, Department of Medicinal Chemistry and Molecular Pharmacology at Purdue University in West Lafayette, Indiana, there are probably more active compounds in SP than we know of at this time. Dr. McLaughlin has personally analyzed some of these compounds at his University laboratory. He says, "There are hundreds of substances in herbal extracts, and it's going to take a very long time for us to isolate the biologically active ones. It's like trying to find a needle in a haystack. For instance, we have isolated two monoglycerides within SP that have anti-tumor activities. These are 1-monolaurin, and 1-monomyristin. I'm sure there are others."

The extracts you buy in vitamin stores, pharmacies, or retail outlets should contain 85% to 95% standardized extract of the fatty acids and sterols ('liposterolic' extracts) found in SP. Unfortunately, not all products will be identical since the extraction process varies from laboratory to laboratory. The final ingredients of the extracts depend on a number of factors. These include which type of solvent is used in the extraction process, the time of year the berries are harvested, the type of soil the palm trees are grown in, and the skill of the technicians at the processing plant.

Dr. McLaughlin strongly believes that the time of year a plant, flower, or berry is picked makes a difference in the content of the active ingredients. "We did a field study collecting paw paw plants (also known as Indiana bananas) every two weeks throughout the year. We found the peak in activity of the compounds to be between May and July. Much of the folkloric use of plants and herbs developed as a consequence of trial and error. Healers learned with time that there were specific periods throughout the year that a particular plant had its most active ingredients.

"Therefore, if a plant is improperly grown, or harvested at an off time, it would either not have the same active ingredients, or have a different set of ingredients that would work in the body a different way."

Almost all of the studies done with SP extracts have used the European trademarked product Permixon (a hexane extract), or Strogen (a carbon dioxide extract). The SP products available over the counter may have liposterolic extracts that are similar to these trademarked products, or perhaps slightly different. If the contents of over-the-counter SP products are different, they may have more active ingredients, or fewer active ingredients. Unfortunately, these are some of the uncertainties needing to be dealt with when using plant extracts that are not fully standardized. Herbal medicine is not yet a pure science.

Berry or Extract?

Some SP products contain crushed berries, rather than the extracts. Until we learn more about the effects of using the full contents of the berries, I recommend using only the extracts. The extracts will contain the actual substances that are effective in treating benign prostate hyperplasia (BPH) in a much higher concentration. The berries provide smaller amounts of the needed active ingredients. Whether the crushed berries have compounds that provide other benefits is not fully known at this time. Use of the berries may require ingesting at least one or two grams a day. The ratio of the dried berry to the lipophilic extracts is usually about 10 to 1. Some users prefer to take both the extracts and the berries, thinking that there are substances within the full berries that could be beneficial. More research is needed.

What About Standardizing SP Products?

Since there are hundreds of substances within SP, it would be difficult to standardize extracts. How can one product be compared to another? Which compounds within SP could serve as markers?

Dr. McLaughlin believes that the monoacylglycerides monolaurin and monomyristin could serve as marker compounds since they are not easily found in other herbs or plants. They could easily be evaluated in a laboratory by a process known as High Performance Liquid Chromatography (HPLC). Thus, by knowing the amounts of these compounds, it would be easier to standardize different products. Beta-sitosterol, one of the plant sterols in SP, may not be a good marker since many other herbs contain this sterol.

St. John's wort is now often standardized by its content of hypericin. For instance, most bottles will say on them that the product contains 0.3 percent hypericin. SP products do not have this standardization, but most bottles will say that they contain 85 to 95 percent of a liposterolic extract. Liposterolic is a general term that encompasses the varieties of fat-soluble compounds within SP.

The standardization of SP products is not likely to occur soon.

Is There a Major Difference Between Different Trademarked Products?

Donald Brown, N.D., the author of *Herbal Prescriptions for Better Health,* (Prima, 1996), and President of Natural Product Research Consultants in Seattle, Washington, says, "The active compounds within SP can be extracted in a variety of ways. The most common is using hexane (a volatile, colorless, liquid hydrocarbon with 6 carbon atoms). The French Company Pierre Fabré Medicaments uses this process for their product Permixon. Another product, called Strogen Forte, contains extracts removed by carbon dioxide. Some vitamin companies will say on their bottle "Non-hexane extract." Frankly, both ways are fine and I don't see any problems with either method of extraction. Hexane is the traditional way to extract fatty acids, oils and sterols from herbs, seeds and berries. Ethanol can also be used for extraction.

"It's possible that the constituents of the different products may be slightly different based on the method of extraction, however, for practical purposes, their effect on the human prostate should not be too different."

I tend to agree with Dr. Brown. For the time being, and for practical purposes, it's okay to consider most of these products as near equivalent.

How Quickly Does SP Get Absorbed?

When you swallow a SP capsule or tablet, it will go into the gastrointestinal tract, be absorbed from the intestines, and make its way to the blood in about an hour or two. The liposterolic extracts have been found to stay in the blood for a few hours. During this time, a number of compounds within the SP extract will make their way to various parts of the body, including skin, hair follicles, genital tissues, and prostate. Studies in rats show that higher concentrations of SP are eventually found in the prostate gland as compared to other tissues (Plosker, 1996).

SP is best taken with meals since it is fat-soluble. Most of the time, the recommended dosage is one 160 mg pill twice a day. However, a dosage of 320 mg taken once a day is also an option.

For What Conditions Is SP Useful?

The best known use of SP is for the treatment of prostate enlargement. However, there's a possibility that substances in SP could have an influence on a variety of body tissues, particularly skin and hair. They may even have anti-tumor potential. A review of the research discussing these influences can be found in Chapter Twelve.

It appears that urinary symptoms resulting from mild-to-moderate prostate enlargement respond more readily to SP than symptoms due to severe enlargement (Ebbinghaus, 1995).

How Does SP Work?

Unfortunately, many herbal and natural medicines have had far less research money devoted to them than they deserve. SP is no exception. Consequently, the answer to the exact mechanisms of how the different compounds within SP work isn't yet known. However, there have been enough studies to give some clues. Some of the most likely mechanisms include the reduction in the amount of dihydrotestosterone (DHT) in prostate tissue, inhibition of the binding of DHT to androgen receptors in prostate cells, and the anti-estrogenic action in prostate tissue. The studies supporting or refuting these claims are discussed in greater detail in a later chapter.

Unlike a particular medicine, such as Proscar, which has only one active ingredient, SP has several different active compounds within it. This complicates the evaluation of all the possible interactions that these compounds have on a variety of tissues within the body. Furthermore, it is possible that a single compound within SP may not have much of an influence on its own although its combination with the other compounds would have a synergistic effect.

The more I learn about the human body, the more I realize how complicated it is. Early in my medical career I often unquestioningly accepted the results of studies done in a laboratory or on animals and was quick to generalize this information to humans. I now know otherwise. In order to understand truly how a medicine works, it has to be studied *directly* on humans. Although laboratory and animal studies can give important information, they are never a replacement for thorough human evaluations.

Another complicating factor is that modern medicine does not advance solely on the basis of seeking the most efficient therapy for human diseases. There are significant economic factors that influence the funding of studies, the subsequent interpretation of the results, and especially the dissemination of this information. Many of the studies done with SP were financed either by companies who market this extract, such as Pierre Fabré Medicament, or by pharmaceutical companies, such as Merck, who have developed competing drugs that treat prostate enlargement. Merck developed the drug Proscar.

The results of studies obtained by Merck scientists on the method of action of SP are often in marked disagreement with the results obtained by scientists working under the auspices of SP-selling companies. (See Chapter Six.)

What About Side Effects?

Various studies and anecdotal evidence indicate that SP is remarkably well tolerated. Only rare instances of side effects have been reported, and usually less than 4% (Descotes, 1995). The most common adverse effects reported in some studies include minor gastrointestinal disorders such as cramps and nausea (Authrie, 1987). These gastrointestinal side effects are minimized when patients take SP with meals. Headaches are infrequent (Champault, 1984). Evaluations of laboratory measurements have not shown SP to have any significant effects on blood studies, kidney function, or liver enzymes (Carraro, 1996).

Any Problems with Long Term Use?

A German study using SP with 315 patients conducted over a three year period, showed prostate symptoms to have improved in 82% of the patients (Bach, 1996). No significant side effects were found and 98 percent of the patients reported tolerating the medicine well. The results of this study are discussed in more detail in Chapter Six.

CHAPTER 3

The Flow is Slow

As people age, their muscles, height, and important organs continue to shrink—except for the prostate gland. It seems to have a mind of its own.

Growing Pains

The majority of older men in North America have an enlarged prostate and a good number of this aging population suffers from symptoms of prostate enlargement, also known as benign prostate hyperplasia (BPH) (Garraway, 1993). Hyperplasia (or hypertrophy) means overgrowth. Since the proportion of elderly people in industrialized nations is increasing, it is quite likely that the prevalence of prostate enlargement will be a more important problem over the coming years.

In addition to annoying older men with urinary problems, the prostate gland can also turn cancerous. Prostate cancer is extremely common, occurring in at least 10 percent of all men in North America. Although not as lethal as lung cancer, it is the second most common non-skin malignancy in males. For older men who have urinary symptoms and discom-

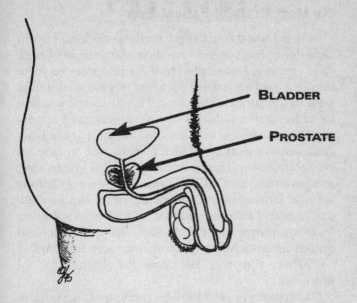

BLADDER

PROSTATE

fort from BPH, it seems that the prostate gland is only good for trouble. However this walnut-sized gland does serve important functions. The prostate is instrumental in adding nutrients and fluid to the sperm. And without well-lubricated sperm, none of us would be here.

The prostate surrounds the beginning part of the urethra and is located right below the urinary bladder (see diagram). The continued enlargement of the prostate results in the narrowing of the passageway from which the urine flows. As the size of this tunnel, known as the urethra, becomes smaller, it becomes more difficult for urine to pass through. There can be times when the problem becomes so severe that urine practically stops coming out.

My Most Grateful Patient Ever

When I was a fourth-year medical student, I spent time doing rotations in various hospital departments. One evening, I was called to the emergency room to admit a patient complaining of severe abdominal pain to the surgical care unit. The suspicion was that he either had a kidney stone or an inflamed appendix. When I walked in the room, the patient was lying restless on a gurney, writhing from side to side, in complete agony. However, his vital signs—heart rate, temperature, and blood pressure—were relatively normal. During the routine taking of the simple medical history, I determined that he had been suffering from symptoms of BPH. In fact, the symptoms had gotten progressively worse over the past few days.

"When did you last visit the bathroom?" I inquired.

"Last night . . . at 9 PM" he replied, while continuing to twist in agony.

"That's more than 22 hours ago," I said, shocked.

"Yea . . . aaah . . . for the past few days my stream has been getting weaker . . . aaah . . . weaker . . . and then it suddenly stopped."

I tapped with the tip of my finger on his lower abdomen. It was obvious that it was swollen and filled with liquid. I asked the nurse to bring me a Foley catheter. I numbed the opening of his urethra and gradually inserted the catheter into it, inch by inch. About eight inches later, there was some resistance. I pushed a little harder . . . and bingo. Urine started coming through the catheter. Within a few minutes, a quart flushed out of his bladder.

"You are great! GREAT! GREAT!" he shouted. I was sure everyone in the adjoining rooms heard him. One of the nurses poked her head through the curtain to see what was going on. He continued, "Next to my wedding day, this is the happiest day of my life!!" After a short pause, and after more urine had come out, he corrected himself. "I take that back. This is THE happiest day of my life!"

The young take for granted that all bodily functions will forever continue working normally. It's only when something starts malfunctioning that attention is paid to the body. I often try to remind myself to be thankful every day that I have my health and am able to enjoy the simple things in life: chewing food and enjoying its taste, walking without any pain, and sleeping without aches.

Some Definitions

Understanding some of the terminology that doctors use when they discuss with their senior patients symptoms associated with prostate enlargement can be useful.

Frequency, meaning frequent urination, can certainly interfere with quality of life. For instance, when a man has to constantly visit the bathroom, he can't take long trips in the car without regular stops. He may, embarrassed, have to excuse himself from boardroom meetings, conversations with people, social gatherings, at the bowling alley, and so on. A person with frequency is not the ideal person to play an 18-hole round at the golf course. The golf-cart trips back to the clubhouse after each hole can surely slow down the game.

Nocturia means urinating frequently during the night. It is basically "frequency" occurring at nighttime. The continued interruptions throughout the night lead to shallow, fragmented sleep and tiredness the next day. The poor sleep quality can even result in low daytime mood or depression. The continued interruptions throughout the night could also disturb the sleep patterns of the spouse if she sleeps in the same room. Sometimes older couples will choose to sleep in different bedrooms because of this problem. Often, the master bedroom with the adjoining bathroom is reserved for the husband to minimize the distance he covers during the night.

Urgency is the feeling of having to go to the bathroom right away. While most young individuals can hold on and wait when they have a full bladder, older individuals with BPH don't have as much control. They can't postpone it. Long car trips can present a problem.

Weak stream means the man now has to step very close to the urinal, or practically be on top of it.

Hesitancy is the term used for dribbling. That is, only small amounts come out of the bladder at any one time. The wait can seem like it is forever, and people start wondering what the heck a man has been doing in the bathroom for the past hour.

Incomplete emptying of the bladder. The leftover urine in the bladder is called **residual volume,** and fertile soup for bacteria to settle, bear offspring, and multiply for many generations, leading to . . .

Cystitis, or bladder infection. Symptoms of cystitis include frequency.

Another symptom of BPH is **dysuria,** meaning painful urination. In addition to BPH, there are many other causes of dysuria including bacterial infections of the bladder or prostate, sexually transmitted diseases, such as gonorrhea and chlamydia, bladder stones, non-infectious prostatitis, or possibly even cancer of the prostate or other organs of the genitourinary system. Surprisingly, SP has been found to be helpful in improving dysuria. A 1995 study of 176 men with BPH showed those given SP in a dose of 160 mg twice daily for one month improved 15% more than those on placebo (Descotes, 1995).

CHAPTER 4

What Causes Prostate Enlargement?

The answers to medical problems should be quite simple and each disease should have one cause and one straightforward cure. Unfortunately, that's not the rule. The human body is incredibly complex, and when it comes to the prostate gland, scientists have not yet fully determined why it enlarges. There are quite a number of factors at play.

Blame the Male Hormones

It is believed that the growth of the prostate gland is greatly influenced by androgens (male hormones), particularly a derivative of testosterone known as dihydrotestosterone (DHT). DHT is made in the testicles and is known to stimulate the growth of the prostate gland. DHT comprises close to 95% of the total androgen content within the nucleus of prostate cells (Bruchovsky, 1971).

Castration, or removal of the testicles, sharply reduces the amount of DHT in the body. It has been known for a long time that when males are surgically castrated, the prostate gland promptly atrophies (shrinks). Men whose testicles have been removed in

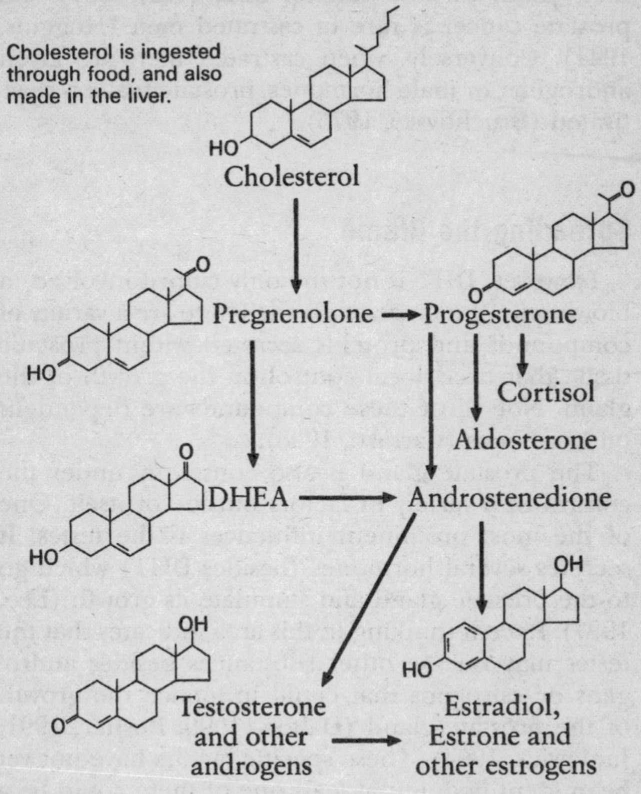

Cholesterol is ingested through food, and also made in the liver.

HO

Cholesterol

Pregnenolone → Progesterone

HO

Cortisol

Aldosterone

DHEA → Androstenedione

HO

OH

HO

Testosterone and other androgens

Estradiol, Estrone and other estrogens

OH

O

Please note that some metabolic steps have been skipped in order to simplify this diagram

METABOLISM OF STEROID HORMONES

Testosterone not only converts to estrogens, but it also converts to dihydrotestosterone (DHT).

their youth do not develop BPH (Wu, 1987) and prostate cancer is rare in castrated men (Huggins, 1941). Conversely, when castrated men are given androgens, or male hormones, prostate tissue is reactivated (Bruchovsky, 1975).

Spreading the Blame

However, DHT is not the only culprit involved in blowing up the prostate gland. There are a variety of compounds and proteins secreted within prostatic tissue that exert local control on the growth of the gland. Not all of these compounds are dependent on hormones (Carraro, 1996).

The prostate gland is also constantly under the control of a variety of factors outside of itself. One of the most prominent influences is the testes. It secretes several hormones (besides DHT) which go to the prostate gland and stimulate its growth (Lee, 1997). Recent thinking in this area indicates that the testes may release other substances besides androgens or estrogens that could influence the growth of the prostate gland (Dalton, 1990; Rosner, 1991; Juniewicz, 1994). These specific factors have not yet been identified, but at least one of them could be a large protein in the blood that transports various hormones. This protein is called steroid hormone-binding globulin (SHBG).

The cause of BPH is not simply an excess of DHT. A variety of local substances within the prostate gland, and a variety of substances or hormones released outside the prostate gland, can also influence its growth. These include the various hormones released from other organs such as the adrenal gland, hypothalamus, and the pituitary (Grayhack, 1963).

That other factors besides androgens influence the growth of the prostate is supported by the fact that while the amount of androgens made by the body declines with age, the prostate gland continues to grow.

Several proteins and growth factors have been identified as possibly influencing the growth of prostate cells (Nishi, 1988; Sherwood, 1992; Desgrandchamps, 1997). The names given to these growth factors include epidermal growth factor (EGF), insulin-like growth factor-I (IGF-I), basic fibroblast growth factor (bFGF), and keratinocyte growth factor (KGF). Recent views about the causes of BPH are changing. Even though androgens may be responsible for the development and functioning of the prostate gland, their effects on growth may be indirect, contingent on their interaction with the above-mentioned growth factors (Desgrandchamps, 1997). This could explain the somewhat disappointing results obtained from the use of Proscar (finasteride). This drug blocks the formation of DHT from testosterone. If DHT is not the only culprit, it would make sense that Proscar is not going to provide full relief of symptoms.

Blame the Female Hormones, Too!

In addition to DHT, and other substances produced from the testicles, there's another hormone possibly involved in enlarging the prostate gland—estrogen, the "female hormone."

There are a number of estrogens including estriol, estradiol, and estrone. Estrogens are believed to stimulate prostate growth, too (Krieg, 1983). In studies with dogs and rat prostate glands, a synergistic effect has been found on prostate growth when both estrogens and androgens are given, compared to just giving androgens (Lee, 1981).

As men age, levels of testosterone in blood decrease while levels of estrogen remain constant, leading to an increase in the ratio of estrogen to androgen in blood and prostate gland (Droller, 1997). In addition, levels of aromatase, an enzyme in the prostate gland responsible for converting androgens to estrogens, increase. Therefore, as men age, the prostate gland becomes exposed to more estrogens. Estrogens are also thought to increase the levels of androgen receptors making them more responsive to the stimulatory effects of testosterone and DHT (Droller, 1997).

The role of estrogens may be due to their ability to stimulate the growth of smooth muscle cells within the prostate gland. These cells are especially prevalent around the urethra, the opening through which urine flows out of the bladder. The enzyme aromatase is most prevalent in the zone of the prostate gland around the urethra. As the muscle cells get larger, or tense up, the urethral opening becomes narrower, making it difficult for urine to come out of the bladder. One type of medicine that is often prescribed to patients with BPH is an alpha-blocker, such as Hytrin. This medicine can relax the smooth muscles, allowing the urine to flow through easier.

In a study done in a laboratory on isolated smooth muscle cells of prostate tissue, the addition of DHT to these muscles stimulated their growth (Zhang, 1997). Interestingly, the addition of estradiol, an estrogen, caused them to grow also, but more dramatically. It appears that, at least on isolated prostate muscle cells, estradiol has more of an effect on the smooth muscle cell growth than does DHT.

It is interesting to speculate that a number of substances in the diet, such as the phytoestrogens (plant estrogens found in soybeans) could have beneficial effects on the prostate gland by acting as weak estrogens and blocking the receptors for the more powerful ones such as estradiol. A number of phytosterols within SP, Pygeum, and other herbs could possibly work in a similar way.

Inflammation as a Cause of BPH

The prostate gland, similar to other organs, can get inflamed. This means that immune cells normally present in the blood can find their way to the gland and irritate it. The reason immune cells would make their way to the prostate could be due to a number of factors. The two most common are:

1. A microorganism, such as a bacteria or virus, has made its way inside the prostate and immune cells are trying to hunt them down (Wright, 1994).
2. Something is going wrong in the prostate, and an autoimmune reaction begins (Theyer, 1992). Cells of the immune system will go there to take care of the problem, however, while doing so, excess amounts of collagen deposition and prostate cell proliferation occurs, leading to BPH.

Blame Your Parents

There may be a genetic factor responsible for BPH. Prostate enlargement is known to run in families. This enlargement may not be due to the role of hormones. When individuals with a family history of BPH were compared to those without BPH, their blood levels of androgens was similar, and both groups responded to Proscar (a medicine that blocks the conversion of testosterone to dihydrotestosterone) in a similar way (Sanda, 1997). The researchers state, "A genetic factor responsible for familiar BPH may exert its influence through androgen independent control of prostate growth."

Blame Your Country

Back in 1936, autopsies were done of prostate glands from Chinese men from Beijing, and compared to autopsies of age-matched men in Western countries (Chang, 1936). The results showed only 6.6 percent of the Chinese men to have had BPH compared to 47 percent of the Westerners. While the incidence of BPH is gradually increasing in Asian countries, it is still less common than in the United States. In 1994, the incidence of BPH in Chinese men was found in one study to be 31 percent (Gu, 1994), while a study in 1984 found 63 percent of American prostates to have BPH (Berry, 1984).

When the prostate glands of Chinese men with BPH are compared to American men, there is a clear difference (Yu, 1997). Chinese prostate tissue samples have higher density of glandular cells compared to American prostates that have a higher percent of connective tissue.

The difference in prostate glands between different races may either be due to genetics, certain unknown environmental factors, or the types of foods eaten.

CHAPTER 5

The Food-Prostate Connection

What is eaten influences every organ of the body. Therefore, it is logical to assume that the prostate gland is responsive to dietary intake.

Benign prostate enlargement and prostate cancer are less common in the Far East than in Western countries (Lee, 1997). Immigrants from China and Japan, after a few generations, begin having a similar incidence of prostate disease as those born and raised in America. This suggests that some environmental factor, probably diet, plays a role in prostate cancer and prostate enlargement (Ekman, 1989).

Although the exact dietary influences on the prostate gland are still being evaluated, many researchers suspect that fruits, vegetables, soy products, and whole grains could provide health benefits to the prostate (Adlercreutz, 1997). Many of these foods contain phytoestrogens, carotenoids, flavonoids, and other plant compounds. Some of these compounds are weak estrogens capable of blocking the effects of stronger estrogens. Flavonoids are known to influence the metabolism of testosterone and other steroid hormones by the liver (Dai, 1997). Over the next few years, specifics on how the various compounds within these foods influence health and the integrity of the prostate gland will be learned.

Have You Chewed on Your Plant Estrogens Today?

Over the past 20 to 30 years, scientists have not only determined the content of many chemicals within plants, but have also evaluated the role of some of these chemicals in health and disease. One group of plant chemicals studied very closely includes the phytoestrogens, or plant estrogens. It has been proposed that the high intake of fat, meats, and sugar in Western diets, along with a lower intake of plant products, could well contribute to the higher rate of cancers in Western Europe and the USA (Adlercreutz, 1997).

The interaction of the thousands of plant chemicals daily consumed with the various tissue systems in the body is extremely complicated. However, it is known that these chemicals not only influence the metabolism of sex hormones, but also influence protein synthesis, cell growth, the health of blood vessels, and have some role to play with practically every organ, tissue, and cell.

Soy products have been very well studied as a source of phytoestrogens. The two best known phytoestrogens within soy are genistein and daidzein. Other plant estrogens include coumestrol, which is found in the highest concentration in mung bean sprouts. Flaxseed (linseed) oil is an abundant source of lignans such as secoisolariciresinol and matairesinol. The examples are indicative of the variety of plant chemicals available in food. Hence, it would be simplistic to recommend one particular plant or vegetable as a "miracle food." They all have important compounds within them that should be consumed. For practical purposes, it's not necessarily important to remember which plant has which type of chemical composition. Men are likely to be on safe ground if they ingest a wide variety of grains, beans, and legumes.

The plant estrogens, when consumed, undergo a number of metabolic conversions in the gut resulting in the formation of hormone-like compounds. These compounds are then absorbed into the bloodstream, enter the tissues, including the prostate gland, and have the ability to bind to estrogen receptors. They can also perform a number of other functions unrelated to their estrogenic effects (Adlercreutz, 1997). For instance, a chemical known as enterolactone (metabolized in the gut from compounds found in flaxseed oil) inhibits the enzyme 5-alpha-reductase. This enzyme converts testosterone to dihydrotestosterone, a hormone partly responsible in stimulating the growth of the prostate gland. Genistein could possibly interfere with some of the growth factors that stimulate the proliferation of prostatic tissue (Linassier, 1989).

The types of foods eaten have more of an influence on the biochemistry of the body than previously imagined.

Lycopene and the Pizza Pie

The carotenoids are plant chemicals responsible for some of the nice colors of produce, such as pink grapefruits, orange apricots, and yellow squash. Hundreds of these carotenoids have been identified. It seems that as soon as a study is published concerning the benefits of one of these plant chemicals, the media turn it into a star. Vitamin companies jump on the bandwagon and make pills containing this particular carotenoid. All the others are temporarily forgotten until a new study is published touting the benefits of the latest carotenoid.

In 1996 and 1997, there was a lot of press about lycopene, a carotenoid found in tomatoes. This was based on the results of a study indicating that intake of this carotenoid reduced the risk of prostate cancer (Giovannucci 1995). Some newspaper or magazine articles have even touted eating more pizza as a way to get additional lycopene and reduce prostate cancer risk. What about the white bread crust, the oil, and all that high-fat cheese? Sometimes reporters and writers simplify things and don't see the overall picture. It's very likely that a number of compounds within vegetables and fruits influence the prostate gland, and focusing on lycopene, at the expense of a complete approach, would be counterproductive.

Should you take lycopene pills? I don't recommend at this time that anyone go out of his way to take this supplement unless he happens to shun tomato products. Americans and Italians normally consume tomatoes, or foods and products containing tomatoes, in greater proportion to other vegetables. I'm concerned that adding high-dose lycopene pills may disturb the balance of other carotenoids and flavonoids in the body. However, if an already available herbal prostate product already includes small amounts of lycopene, I think it's fine to take these pills.

Baffled by Beta-Carotene

An article appeared in the July 15, 1997 issue of *Family Practice News* reporting new data from the Physicians' Health Study, which showed the relationship between intake of beta-carotene and prostate cancer to be quite complex.

The Physicians' Health Study is funded by The National Cancer Institute. The study began in 1982 when 22,071 male physicians were randomized to receive either beta-carotene or placebo and were followed in a double-blind fashion for 12 years. Men who had very low levels of beta-carotene at the start of the study had a reduction of prostate cancer when they took 50,000 units of beta-carotene a day. However, men who had higher than normal levels of beta-carotene in their blood at the start of the study had a higher rate of prostate cancer if they took supplements of beta-carotene. These results were reported by Dr. Meir Stampfer at the annual meeting of the American Society of Clinical Oncology. Dr. Stampfer is Professor of Epidemiology and Nutrition at the Harvard School of Public Health in Boston.

A close look at the data showed that men who initially had low levels of beta-carotene, indicating a low intake of fruits and vegetables, had a 36 percent greater rate of cancer at all sites compared to men with the highest level of initial beta-carotene. Since levels of beta-carotene often reflect a person's fruit and vegetable consumption, these results are consistent with various other studies that testify fruits and vegetables protect against cancer.

Even though men with low beta-carotene levels benefited from supplements, I prefer that they get this carotenoid from dietary sources instead of from a pill. The reason for the increased rate of prostate cancer in individuals with higher levels of beta-carotene who also supplemented with beta-carotene is that excessive intake of this carotenoid may have caused an imbalance. Normally hundreds of carotenoids are ingested on a daily basis. By taking too much of one carotenoid, an imbalance or relative deficiency of another carotenoid within our tissues and cells may be caused.

It's quite easy to get adequate amounts of plant chemicals if a few pieces of fruits, vegetables, grains, and legumes are consumed on a daily basis. Drinking a few ounces of vegetable or fruit juices a day is also acceptable, though it is preferable these juices be a mix of a few different types in order to get a variety of different plant chemicals.

Green Tea Anyone?

A popular drink in the Orient is green tea. It is possible this tea may play a role in the lower incidence of prostate problems in Asians. Green tea is known to contain many antioxidants and is also thought to have compounds which act as 5-alpha-reductase inhibitors (Liao, 1995).

Let's Cut to the Fat

With all the research that has been done over the years, a clearer idea on whether, or if, fat is involved with prostate cancer should be known. At least one study has shown a very good association between intake of fat, especially saturated fat, and the risk of developing aggressive prostate cancer (West, 1991). But, a true scientist does not come to quick conclusions until there is a preponderance of evidence.

Such a scientist is Dr. L.N. Kolonel, of the Epidemilology Program at the University of Hawaii in Honolulu. In a 1996 article published in *Cancer Causes Control*, Dr. Kolonel says,

The role of fat in prostate cancer remains unclear. Few studies, to date, have adjusted the results for caloric intake, and no particular fat component has been consistently implicated. A notable finding is a strong positive association with intake of animal products, especially red meats, but this in itself does not specifically implicate fat.

It will take a long time to have enough evidence to convince hard-core scientists on the relationship of fat to prostate cancer. In the meantime, eating fewer greasy hamburgers and substituting fish appears to be wise.

Palatable Paths to a Petite Prostate

Even with all these uncertainties, I am willing to make some preliminary recommendations until more evidence accumulates. For a healthier body and prostate:

1. Increase intake of fresh fruits and vegetables. Beta-carotene or lycopene supplements are not necessary if a few pieces of vegetables and fruits are consumed each day; or mixed juices are drunk.
2. If excessive calories from fats are currently consumed, decrease intake to 20 to 30 percent or so of calories.
3. Include fat from fish, or fish oils in the diet. A small amount of flaxseed oil may be beneficial.
4. Incorporate more legumes and grains in the diet. They contain phytoestrogens and lignans.

5. Soy products are a great choice. They contain phytosterols, or phytoestrogens, such as genistein. Reduce tobacco and alcohol consumption. Excessive alcohol intake has shown to be toxic to rat prostates (Novelli, 1997).
6. Reduce intake of sugar and calories.
7. Substitute herbal teas for sodas and sugared drinks. There are dozens of different types of herbal teas in grocery or health food stores. Buy half a dozen or so different ones and each morning try something new. Enjoy green tea. Herbal teas can be sweetened with a natural, non-caloric sweetener called stevia.

CHAPTER 6

The Incredible Shrinking Prostate? The Science of SP

Pharmaceutical companies have provided us with some wonderful medicines. So has nature. Pharmaceutical companies have, at times, also marketed dangerous drugs. Nature has also created dangerous herbs and plants. I often hear people emphatically claiming that herbal therapies are safe and are preferable to drugs. Although this is generally true, it would be simplistic to unequivocally assert that substances found in nature are inherently safer and superior to those synthesized in laboratories. Each chemical, whether natural or man-made, has to be evaluated on its own merit. During the millions of years of evolution, plants have created chemicals to help them not only extract and use nutrients found in soil, water, and air, but also chemicals to make themselves unpalatable and toxic to insects and animals bent on consuming them. Poisonous Amanita mushrooms are a case in point. Many chemicals found in plants and herbs are not fit for human consumption. The only good way to find out the medicinal merits of a particular herb is to do extensive short-term and long-term human testing.

Certain plants produce chemicals that are beneficial for human consumption. Examples are fruits and vegetables. Not only do they contain carbohydrates, fats, proteins, vitamins, and minerals, but they also have thousands of nutrients including bioflavonoids and carotenoids that, fortunately, have enormous health-promoting properties. Additionally, many plants have been found to have chemicals that have potential in the therapy of a variety of human ailments, including fighting infections and tumors. SP is one such plant. It contains compounds that have a beneficial influence on the human prostate gland.

The Proof is In the Flow

One of the earliest studies evaluating the role of SP in the therapy of BPH was done in 1984 by Dr. Champault and colleagues at the Hospital Jean Verdier in Bondy, France. These researchers used a trademarked version of SP extract named Permixon, which is owned by a French company called Pierre Fabré Medicaments. (Other trademarks include Capistan, Strogen, Libeprosta and Sereprostat.) Permixon's main components are free (90%) and esterified (7%) fatty acids, sterols, flavonoids and other substances (Carraro, 1996).

Fifty-five patients with BPH who had symptoms of frequent urination, nocturia, and poor urinary flow were given 160 mg of Permixon twice a day for 30 days. The results were compared to another group who received placebo pills. At the end of this period, both objective measurements of urinary flow and subjective reporting from patients had improved on average by 50 percent compared to placebo. The medicine was well tolerated with only minor side effects reported, one being headaches. Standard blood chemistry measurements showed no changes.

The researchers conclude, "As predicted from pharmacological and biochemical studies, Permixon appears to be a useful therapeutic tool in the treatment of benign prostatic hyperplasia."

It should be noted that many of the studies evaluating the effects of SP were conducted or funded by the pharmaceutical company that sells Permixon, the trademarked version of SP extract.

Champault and colleagues published a follow up study that involved administering Permixon to 47 patients with prostatic adenoma. An adenoma is a benign growth or cancer that has a very low risk of spreading or expanding. The study period this time went for 14 months, and in some cases up to two and a half years. They found the medicine to be efficacious and perfectly tolerated (Champault, Bonnard, 1984).

Two years later, a British group headed by Dr. Reece Smith, from the Department of Urology and Radiology at Southampton General Hospital, repeated a similar study. Thirty-three patients were given Permixon at 160 mg twice daily and compared to a group of 37 individuals who did not receive any therapy. Interestingly, both the medication treated group and the placebo group had a significant improvement in flow rate and symptoms. No side effects were noted on Permixon except for two patients who had nausea, and one who reported an increase in sexual drive. The researchers did not seem to be completely convinced of SP's benefits. They say, "In conclusion, whilst the regime of Permixon used in this trial was safe, well tolerated and associated with considerable, symptomatic improvement, we have no evidence that this improvement was due to anything more than the psychosocial value of being involved in the trial and meeting a number of sufferers from a similar condition."

With these conflicting reports on the effectiveness of SP, an extensive study was sorely needed. Fortunately, such a study was published in 1996. Not only did it evaluate the effectiveness of SP in the therapy of BPH, but it also compared this herb to Proscar, the medical gold standard in the therapy of BPH.

Herb vs. Drug—The Match of the Decade

The big contest had come with billions of future dollars riding on the outcome. Could extracts from a common, dwarf palm tree berry compete with the so-called "gold standard" of traditional BPH therapy? Merck and Company, one of the largest pharmaceutical corporations in the world, had invested hundreds of millions of dollars in the past decade in creating, studying, and marketing finasteride (Proscar). This medicine has become one of the most frequently used drugs in the therapy of BPH. But, could there be a cheaper, as effective, and more natural alternative?

The largest study ever done comparing Proscar with SP was a six month double-blind, randomized trial organized by Pierre Fabré Medicaments and it included 1,098 men (Carraro, 1996). Double blind means that neither the researchers, nor the patients, know whether they are taking the real medicine or a dummy pill until the code is broken at the end of the study. It was done in 87 urology centers in nine European countries. All the men had BPH, were over the age of 50 years, and had symptoms associated with bladder flow obstruction.

SP extract, in the form of the trademarked version Permixon, was administered at a dose of 160 mg twice a day, in the morning and evening, for a period of 26 weeks. This was compared to Proscar at a 5 mg dosage in the morning. Each patient was evaluated prior to the start of the medicines, at 6 weeks, 13 weeks, and after 26 weeks. At each of these visits, urinary flow rates were measured, an International Prostate Symptom Score (IPSS) was determined, and each patient was requested to complete a form evaluating their quality of life, including their sexual function. The IPSS had seven questions relating to urgency, daytime and nighttime urinary frequency, hesitancy, sensation of incomplete voiding, and force of urine stream.

Ultrasound examinations of the bladder were done at 13 and 26 weeks to evaluate the amount of urine left in the bladder as well as to assess the size of the prostate gland. Several blood studies were also done, including measuring prostate specific antigen (PSA) levels. High PSA levels are often indicative of prostate cancer.

Who Won?

It was a close tie with both medicines showing advantages and disadvantages. Both SP and Proscar similarly decreased the total IPSS score. There was improvement noted in both groups within 6 weeks, and the improvement continued as the study went on. Other findings included:

Prostate size—both medicines reduced the size of the prostate gland, however, Proscar was more effective with a 16% reduction versus SP at only 7%.

Quality of life—more than half of the patients in both groups felt their quality of life had improved after 6 weeks of treatment and 70% reported improvement by 26 weeks. Both treatment regimens were thus comparable.

Sexual function—only one patient in each treatment group withdrew from the study because of sexual problems. However, patients on Proscar reported a slight deterioration in sexual function compared to those on SP. They had a higher incidence of decreased libido, impotence, and ejaculatory disorders.

Urinary flow—the ability to urinate rapidly improved in both groups with a slightly higher improvement on Proscar

Residual volume—the amount of urine left in the bladder increased by 8 ml with SP and decreased by 4 ml with Proscar.

Acute urinary retention—seven patients on SP and three patients on Proscar had to be hospitalized due to worsening of symptoms and the inability to urinate.

The researchers conclude, "The results of this double-blind randomized study demonstrate that 320 mg daily of Permixon and 5 mg of finasteride are equally effective in the management of BPH. Unpublished observations suggest that Permixon is as active as finasteride on medium-sized and small prostates, but is less inhibitory on very large prostates. This difference might be at the origin of the higher incidence of urinary retention we noted with Permixon in this study.

"In the treatment of men with mild or moderate symptoms of BPH, Permixon and finasteride are clinically equivalent. The long-term efficacy of finasteride has been established in placebo-controlled studies; that of Permixon needs to be confirmed."

The results of this trial were presented at the Third International Consultation on BPH held in Monaco in June of 1995. A great amount of discussion between the presenting panel and experts in the audience was generated. Skeptics complained that the trial period of 26 weeks was not long enough to come to any firm conclusions. In an accompanying editorial in the same journal, *The Prostate*, Dr. L. J. Denis, from the Department of Urology at Algemeen Ziekenhrs Middelheim in Belgium, did not yet seem completely convinced since the study did not include a placebo group. It is known that the placebo effect is quite high in the therapy of BPH. Dr. Denis concludes, as practically every scientist does when asked what to make of the results of a study, "We hope to see more randomized trials in the near future confirming or refuting the data obtained in this trial."

The Longest Study

Although doctors have used SP with patients for over a decade, an actual study evaluating the long-term use of this herb was not published until 1996 (Bach, 1996).

This was a trial conducted in Germany, where doctors have been using SP and other herbs for the therapy of BPH on a regular basis for many years. A total of 89 urologists and 435 patients entered the 3-year prospective study and 315 patients completed it. The patients' age ranged between 41 and 89 years. They were treated with SP at 160 mg twice a day for 3 years.

The results showed nocturia to be improved in 73 percent of the patients. At the start of the study, only 13 patients did not have nocturia, whereas, at the conclusion of the 3-year trial, 114 patients were symptom-free. Daytime frequency improved in 54 percent of the patients. Residual volume diminished by 50 percent. With respect to digital rectal examination, after three years of therapy with SP, no changes in the size of the prostate could be determined.

Overall, 80 percent of the patients and doctors felt the improvements on SP were either good or very good. The researchers conclude, "If one compares the results of the present three-year study of IDS 89 (SP extract) with published data on the long-term treatment of BPH using synthetic active ingredients—i.e., a three-year finasteride study (Stone, 1994), and an 18-months study on the selective alpha-1-blocker, terazosin (Wilde, 1993)—one can, despite methodological reservations, conclude somewhat unexpectedly that better clinical efficacy [effectiveness] has been documented in respect to the herbal preparation. Withdrawal from therapy because of adverse events was 1.8 percent with SP, as opposed to 11 percent with finasteride and 10 percent with terazosin."

This study is very important because it has been known that patients with BPH have a significant response to placebo that can go on for many months, even up to two years. This finding was reported by Dr. J. Curtis Nickel, professor or urology at Queen's University Faculty of Medicine in Kingston, Ontario, at the 1997 annual meeting of the American Urological Association (*Family Practice News,* August 1, 1997, p. 30). Therefore, the 3-year study reported above lends additional credence to the effectiveness of SP. Unfortunately, this 3-year study was not placebo-controlled. Hence, more long-term, placebo-controlled studies are required to satisfy the skepticism of critics.

The Very Latest

A Hungarian study published in 1997 is the latest to show the effectiveness of SP (Kondas, 1997). Thirty-eight patients with symptoms of BPH were given SP for a 12-month period. Nearly three fourths of the patients reported improvements, and no side effects were observed. According to studies measuring the urine flow, the peak flow rate (how fast the urine comes out of the bladder) increased significantly and the amount of urine left in the bladder decreased or was nil in nine out of the ten patients. The size of the prostate gland decreased by 10 percent. The researchers say, "On the basis of this favorable experience, the authors recommend the administration of SP extract in the treatment of patients with mild or moderate symptoms of prostatic hyperplasia."

Summary

The results of numerous studies published over the past 15 or so years indicate that SP improves symptoms in a reasonable number of patients suffering from BPH. The benefits occur often without a dramatic decrease in the size of the prostate gland. The response to SP is similar in many ways to that of Proscar, even though they probably work in different ways.

CHAPTER 7

How Does SP Work?

Over the past few years I have read quite a number of articles published in consumer health magazines on SP, talked to a number of doctors who use it, and followed some of the discussions on the internet on this topic. One thing that seems to be consistent is the general lack of understanding of the complexity of how SP actually works. Many people seem to have the simple idea that SP functions by blocking the conversion of testosterone to DHT.

It is often difficult to determine the exact cause of action of a particular herbal or plant extract since there are a variety of chemicals within this extract that would have a number of different effects in the body. This is particularly true of SP extract since it has many fatty acids, fatty alcohols, phytosterols, and other compounds. It is quite likely that SP extracts function by a multitude of ways. Not all the mechanisms are understood yet. However, over the years, a number of studies have been done that give us some clues. The following are some of the proposed mechanisms of how SP reduces symptoms of prostate enlargement (Plosker, 1996).

- Inhibiting the conversion of testosterone to dihydrotestosterone (DHT).
- Inhibition of binding of DHT to adrogen receptors in prostate cells.
- Blocking the effect of estrogen on prostate tissue.
- Inhibition of growth factors responsible for stimulation of prostate tissue.

A discussion of each of these mechanisms, and others, with supporting or refuting evidence first requires an explanation of how hormones are metabolized in prostate tissue.

A Few Words about Androgens

Testosterone is the best-known androgen, or male hormone. It is made primarily by the testicles, ovaries, and adrenal glands. Once testosterone is made, it can act locally or enter the bloodstream to travel to all parts of the body. Testosterone can have an influence on a variety of organs including skin, hair, brain, muscles, liver, and heart.

The enzyme 5-alpha-reductase converts testosterone to a more potent androgen known as dihydrotestosterone (DHT). This enzyme is present in a variety of body tissues, but not evenly. Some tissues, such as hair, skin and prostate have an active 5-alpha-reductase enzyme and are able to efficiently convert testosterone into DHT. Other tissues, such as muscle, cannot easily convert testosterone into DHT.

DHT is one of the culprits responsible for prostate gland enlargement, acne, male pattern baldness and, in women, excessive hair growth in unwanted places (Tenover, 1991). There is an inherited enzyme deficiency that occurs in humans which has given us clues on what happens when DHT is not formed. There are reports from the Dominican Republic and Turkey of certain families that have males who have a genetic deficiency. They can't make DHT. Blood studies show low levels of DHT while their blood testosterone levels are high.

All females affected with this condition appear normal. Males have problems: they are born with undefined genitalia, a small penis, and testicles that don't descend. Fortunately for them, at puberty, their blood testosterone levels rise, their penis enlarges and the testicles descend. Even more fortunate is that they have no acne, little hair growth on their bodies, no prostate enlargement, and no receding hairline!

This genetic enzyme deficiency of 5-alpha-reductase, and the subsequent absence of DHT, gives enormous clues to the function of this hormone. It suggests that medicines that block the conversion of testosterone to DHT, or block the influence of DHT on certain tissues such as hair, skin and prostate, may not be such a bad thing after all. Joyce Tanover, M.D., Assistant Professor of Medicine at Emory University School of Medicine in Atlanta, Georgia, says, "It is of interest that at least three of the major effects of DHT in the postpubertal male are in areas that are considered to be undesirable or to lead to a 'disease'; namely, prostate growth, acne, and baldness. It is not surprising that such information has led to a search for effective and specific human 5-alpha-reductase inhibitors. Such compounds might be useful in the treatment of acne, BPH, or male pattern baldness and are potentially without major adverse effects."

Keeping in mind that these are theories, not definite answers, we'll look in more detail at some potential ways on how SP can help reduce prostatic symptoms.

Inhibiting the Conversion of Testosterone to DHT

As previously discussed, one of the causes of BPH is the influence of DHT on prostate cells. If the levels of DHT can be decreased within prostate tissue, there is a good chance the gland will shrink enough to allow urine to flow out easier. Can SP block the conversion of testosterone to DHT?

It depends on which laboratory is doing the study. In 1993, scientists at Merck Research Laboratory in Rahway, New Jersey, after evaluating Proscar and SP on rat prostate tissue, concluded that SP does not have the ability to block the conversion of testosterone to DHT while finasteride (Proscar) does (Rhodes, 1993). A year later, a research group from Hôpital Universitaire Cochin, in Paris, determined that the administration of SP extract for a one-week period to 32 healthy male volunteers did not reduce DHT levels in blood; but Proscar administration at 5 mg a day did reduce blood DHT levels (Strauch, 1994). Merck which sells Proscar, funded this study as well.

The findings by Merck researchers conflict with earlier studies financed by the company promoting Permixon which found that SP did have the ability to block the conversion of testosterone to DHT (Briley, 1984).

Many individuals now have easy access to Medline and other medical data information systems through their computer. For instance, if someone wanted to find out more about SP, they would type in saw palmetto or *Serenoa repens* and abstracts of studies on this herbal extract would show on the screen. What doesn't appear within the abstract, but is mentioned in the full article published in a journal, is who is funding the study. What's disturbing is that doctors, the media, or anyone who wants to learn more about SP, or any other supplement, won't realize that some of the information they are reading may not be completely accurate. The results of a particular study may be influenced by the source of the funding.

Dr. Franco Di Silverio and colleagues, from the University of La Sapienza in Rome, Italy, wanted to find out the effect of finasteride (Proscar) and SP on the concentrations of DHT in prostate tissue. Six patients were given SP extract (Permixon) at 320 mg/day for 3 months, 9 patients were given finasteride, and 9 patients were not given any medicines. Prostate tissue was removed surgically from these patients at the conclusion of the three months and levels of DHT were evaluated. In the untreated group, DHT levels were 1121 mg/pg DNA (pg means picogram, one trillionth of a gram). Patients on finasteride showed a level of 232, while those on SP had levels of 256. This study indicates that both finasteride and SP extracts have the ability to decrease DHT levels in prostate tissue. More studies are needed to confirm these findings.

Interestingly, SP does not seem to influence levels of testosterone in the blood. When twenty men, aged 50 to 75 years, suffering from BPH were given 160 mg of SP extract twice a day for one month, there were no changes in their blood levels of testosterone, follicle-stimulating hormone, and luteinizing hormone (Casarosa, 1988).

To make things more conflicting, an additional

study was published by researchers at the Endocrine Unit of Szent-Gyorgyi Albert Medical University, in Szeged, Hungary (Toth, 1996). An SP extract, called Strogen forte was found to inhibit prostatic 5-alpha-reductase in rats and humans.

I have read quite a number of articles on SP in the last few years in lay magazines. Almost every one of the authors reports that the mechanism of action of SP is due to its blocking the conversion of testosterone to DHT. Based on the review of all the studies published thus far, I cannot come to a definite determination on whether compounds within SP block the conversion of testosterone to DHT. It would be premature to make this claim. The results of independently funded studies are needed.

Preventing the Binding of DHT to Androgen Receptors in Prostate Cells

After DHT is converted from testosterone, it has the ability to go to the prostate cell, attach to the DNA, and influence it to make specific enzymes and proteins. This could lead to prostatic growth. One of the presumed ways SP could work is by attaching itself to the DHT receptor on the prostate cell membrane, or somewhere inside the prostate cell thus preventing the action of DHT (Carilla, 1984). This could be compared to trying to open the door of a house with the key but a neighborhood teenager has played a trick. He has filled the hole with a piece of gum. The key is unable to enter the keyhole, and the door won't open.

In a study conducted at the Department of Obstetrics and Gynecology at King Khalid University Hospital in Riyadh, Saudi Arabia, Permixon (the lipid extract of SP) was dissolved in 9 different tissues of human tissue specimens (Mgdy El-Sheikh, 1988). These included uterine, vaginal skin, abdominal wall skin, and skin from circumcised babies. In all of the specimens, SP was able to block DHT receptors by about 40 percent. The researchers stated, "Since hirsutism [excessive hair growth on the face and body, especially in women] and virilism [masculinization] are among gynecological problems caused either by excessive androgen stimulation or excess end organ response, we suggest that Permixon could be a useful treatment in such conditions and recommend further investigations of the possible therapeutic values of the drug in gynecological practice."

Whether SP will have a role to play in acne, hair loss, or other conditions associated with excessive androgen stimulation, has not been fully determined at this time.

Blocking the Effect of Estrogen on Prostate Tissue

There are quite a number of receptors within the prostate gland for androgens, such as testosterone, and likewise quite a number for estrogens. Scientists are starting to suspect that excessive amounts of estrogens influence the growth of the prostate gland. There is at least one study that found SP to have anti-estrogenic abilities within prostate tissue.

A double-blind, placebo-controlled study was done with 35 patients with BPH who had never before been treated with any medicines (Di Silverio, 1992). Eighteen of these patients received 160 mg SP extract a day for 3 months and were compared to 17 others who received placebo pills. At the end of the study, prostatic tissue was surgically removed and evaluated for hormone receptors. SP extract was able to inhibit not only androgen receptors, but also estrogen receptors. The researchers conclude, "This drug, therefore, appears to display an inhibitory effect both on androgen receptors and estrogen receptors, probably because it is composed by several fractions, one of which with anti-androgenic action and another with anti-estrogenic action. . . . The inhibition of the estrogen action may be applied to the treatment of BPH, since there is increasing evidence that the primary role of androgens in the genesis of the disease may be conditioned by other factors, one of these being estrogens. . . . So, one may assume that in the medical treatment of human BPH, inhibition of the estrogen action potentiates [enhances] the effects of the anti-androgens."

Inhibition of Growth Factors Responsible for Stimulation of Prostate Tissue

In addition to the above mentioned possibilities involved in the growth of the prostate gland, a number of growth factors previously mentioned have a role to play in BPH. These include epidermal growth factor (EGF), fibroblast growth factor (FGF), and others (Paubert Braquet, 1995). SP may play a role in the function of these growth factors.

And More Ways

There may be other ways that extracts from SP could influence the prostate gland. These include:

- Preventing the action of the hormone prolactin from stimulating prostatic growth (Vacher, 1995). Prolactin is a hormone secreted by the pituitary gland in the brain. It is best known for stimulating the secretion of milk and possibly, during pregnancy, stimulating breast growth.
- Preventing inflammation of prostate cells by inhibiting the production of prostaglandins and arachidonic acid (Ragab, 1987). Prostaglandins are a class of biologically active substances present in many tissues (first found in genital fluids and prostate gland, hence the name) that mediate inflammatory and immune reactions. Arachidonic acid is a precursor to prostaglandins and is involved in inflammation. These factors may be of importance since it is believed that inflammation of the prostate sometimes precedes the hormonally induced proliferation of prostate tissue (Robinette, 1988).
- In one study conducted on rodents, a lipid extract from SP was able to have relaxing effects on the rat uterus (Gutilerrez, 1996). It is interesting to note that, in the 1800s, some women were given SP berries for certain gynecological problems, including painful periods. Painful periods can sometimes result from spasms of the uterine muscle tissue. Is there a connection? How this information can be translated into practical human terms is currently unknown. Since part of the symptoms of prostate enlargement are due to muscle spasm around the bladder neck, decreasing the flow from the bladder, could reducing the spasms improve the flow of urine? This possibility is purely theoretical and based on minimal evidence. However, it's interesting to keep in mind that perhaps, in the future,

we will find SP extracts to have other medical benefits in both men and women. Compounds within SP may have other influences on our physiology that we currently are not aware.

- Dr. Jerry McLaughlin, from Purdue University, has another thought. He tells me, "We have found that certain monoacylglycerides in SP have the ability to be incorporated into cell membranes and break open the cell membrane, thus killing the cell. Since many of these monoacylglycerides are specific for prostate cells, could [the] shrinking of the prostate gland be due to [the] destruction of prostate cells [by the monoacylglycerides in SP]?"

Prostate enlargement has many causes and it will take a long time to find out how SP works in helping individuals with symptoms of prostate enlargement. For the latest updates, see website www.raysahelian. com or subscribe to *Longevity Research Update* (see last pages of book).

CHAPTER 8

How is SP Available?

The majority of the studies done with SP have used a proprietary brand called Permixon, available in Europe, which contains 160 mg of SP extract. As a consequence, most of the vitamin companies marketing SP in the States have also chosen to include 160 mg in their capsules.

There is no reason that the pills have to contain exactly 160 mg. It's just the dosage a company called Pierre Fabré Medicaments picked many years ago in order to standardize their formulation. It's likely that a range of dosages, possibly anywhere from 100 mg to 200 mg twice daily, would work. However, excessive doses are not necessarily more effective. In a study done in Germany, 49 patients were randomized to receive either 160 mg of SP twice daily or 480 mg twice daily. After a 6 month trial, both groups were found to have similar benefits (Dathe, 1991). It's theoretically possible that a higher dose of SP taken initially for a week or two may provide quicker benefits. No studies have been published evaluating this option. I know one physician who recommends patients initially start on 360 mg 3 times per day for a week and then lower the dosage to 160 mg twice a day.

Products Available Over the Counter

Since SP cannot be patented, there are hundreds of vitamin companies that sell it. The majority will provide capsules of 160 mg of SP liposterolic extract. The percentage of the liposterolic extract, in most cases, will be listed as 85 to 95 percent.

Most brands of SP offered by local vitamin or retail stores, or mail order catalogs, contain 160 mg per capsule or tablet. Some will have 80 mg, requiring ingestion of two of these capsules, twice daily. Some contain 320 mg. Once a day dosing should be sufficient with these.

Since the active ingredients in SP are fat soluble, it is uncertain that teas containing extracts of this herb would provide enough of the liposterols and fatty acids to be effective. Therefore, for the time being, do not exclusively rely on the teas as a complete source for the active compounds.

A thorough search of local vitamin stores or pharmacies, will produce a wide range of dosages, along with SP in combination with other herbs. A recent investigation of some vitamin stores in the Los Angeles area revealed the following:

- SP 80 mg per capsule
- SP 160 mg
- SP 320 mg
- SP 350 mg
- SP 160 mg with 10 mg of zinc
- SP 100 mg with Pygeum 50 mg
- SP 80 mg with raw prostate
- Two tablets provide SP 160 mg, Pygeum 10 mg, pumpkin seed extract 500 mg, lycopene 500 mcg, beta-sitosterol 25 mg, zinc 5 mg, lutein 500 mcg, curcumin (turmeric extract) 50 mg

- Two tablets provide SP 100 mg, Pygeum 100 mg and parsley 75 mg.
- Four capsules provide SP 320 mg, Pygeum 100 mg of 13 percent total sterols
- Saw palmetto complex of 80 mg, pumpkin seed oil extract, cucurbita pepo at 40 mg, Pygeum africanum at 10 mg with 13 percent total sterols, and Bearberry (Uva ursi) at 5 mg containing 10 percent arbutin.

This sampling shows there are quite a number of products on the market with countless combinations of SP along with different amounts of herbs, minerals, and nutrients. The most important factor to look for is the amount of SP present within the capsule since SP is the most well studied herb in the therapy of prostate gland enlargement. The second most important herb to consider is Pygeum. Also, make sure the bottle says "Guaranteed to contain 85 to 95 percent phytosterols."

Some of the other herbs can be very helpful, too. These are discussed in Chapter Nine. Chapter Fifteen summarizes an approach to take when starting an herbal prostate program.

One of the above products contains raw prostate. I don't see any reason why raw prostate would be important to ingest. The bottle doesn't even list where the raw prostate came from. Stay away from any product that includes raw prostate in its formulation.

The majority of the bottles contain 60 capsules, a month's supply if taking one capsule of 160 mg SP twice daily. As a rule, the cost of SP is less than the cost of pharmaceutical pills that treat prostate enlargement. But be careful about buying some of the combination products since they may not include enough SP.

Sometimes a particular product seems relatively inexpensive compared to another one, but, a closer examination reveals that two or more capsules must be ingested to equal one capsule of another product. For instance, one of the products listed above has 30 pills per bottle and two tablets provide 160 mg of SP. Therefore, at 4 pills a day, the bottle won't even last 8 days! This is also true of certain multivitamin products where I've sometimes read that one has to consume 4 tablets three times a day to get the amount of ingredients listed on the label.

I've seen another product that may mislead you in terms of dosage. On the front of the label, it says that the capsule contains 320 mg of SP. However, at the side of the label, it states that it actually only has 160 mg of SP mixed in an olive oil base of 160 mg, half the dosage listed on the front. Always read all the words on a label. If unsure, ask the pharmacist or the vitamin store manager.

CHAPTER 9

Herbs and Nutrients for a Happy Prostate

Medical doctors in the United States are quite behind when it comes to taking advantage of the therapeutic potential of herbal products. Various herbs and herbal extracts have been approved in European countries, such as Germany and France, for the treatment of a variety of diseases. Fortunately, things are changing in this country. More and more doctors are realizing that nutrients and herbs have a significant role to play in health and disease. Doctors are starting to combine both drug and natural modalities in their practice. In fact, many European researchers feel that the future of medicine may lie in finding the most effective way of combining herbs and drugs (Vahlensieck, 1996).

My main discussion thus far has been on the use of SP for BPH. However, other herbs, plants, and extracts have also been studied for their therapeutic potential (Fitzpatrick, 1995). In Germany, many of these phytopharmaceuticals (plant medicines) have been approved by the government for the therapy of BPH. In addition to SP, some of these include Pygeum africanum, pumpkin seeds, Stinging nettle root, and Rye pollen extract (Vahlensieck, 1996). I'll discuss the latest research with these and other herbs along with a review of nutrients that play a role in the health of the prostate gland.

Pygeum africanum is a large evergreen tree found in central and southern Africa. The extracts from its bark contain several compounds thought to be helpful in reducing prostate enlargement. These include beta-sitosterol, other plant estrogens, triterpenes, and certain compounds known as ferulic acids.

Pygeum extracts have been used for more than 25 years in France for patients suffering from prostate enlargement (Paubert-Braquet, 1994). One trademarked name for Pygeum is Tadenan.

In 1990, a double-blind, placebo-controlled study was done in France, Germany, and Austria with 263 patients (Barlet, 1990). Double blind means that neither the researchers, nor the patients, know whether they are taking the real medicine or a dummy pill until the code is broken at the end of the study. This assures that a patient's expectations do not influence the results of the study.

Capsules of 50 mg of Pygeum africanum extract or placebo were given at a dosage of one capsule in the morning and one in the evening for a period of 60 days. Treatment with this extract led to a marked improvement in the ability to urinate easily. The ones who got the Pygeum improved by 66 percent while those on placebo improved by 31 percent. The only side effects were gastrointestinal symptoms that occurred in only 5 out of the 263 patients.

To test the influence of Pygeum on sexual behavior, a clinical study was designed to give twice the normal dose of Pygeum to patients with prostate enlargement (Carani, 1991). For a period of 60 days, 18 patients were given 200 mg of Pygeum (instead of 100 mg) a day. Symptoms of BPH improved in the patients and no side effects were reported. Interestingly, there was an improvement in sexual behavior in the men.

Which is more effective, SP or Pygeum? A study comparing the two has been done. In a placebo-controlled trial done back in 1983, 60 patients received 320 mg a day of SP and compared to another group that received Pygeum (Mandressi, 1983). The study lasted one month. There was significantly greater improvement with SP than with Pygeum. Keep in mind, that each extract could work in a different way and perhaps the combination of both would have a synergistic effect. Many over-the-counter products combine both of these medicines.

The exact mechanism of how Pygeum influences the prostate gland is currently not known. As with many other extracts, a variety of compounds within Pygeum could work together for a synergistic effect. One possible explanation is Pygeum's ability to display anti-inflammatory activity within prostate cells (Marconi, 1986). As discussed in an earlier chapter on the causes of prostate enlargement, infiltration by immune cells is one of the reasons for BPH. In one study done in France, extracts of Pygeum were found to inhibit infiltration of prostate tissue by immune cells (Paubert-Braquet, 1994).

A most recent study published in 1997 evaluated the role of a Pygeum extract in relation to growth (or proliferation) of prostate cells, specifically the growth of fibroblasts (Yablonsky, 1997). Fibroblasts are large, oval cells found in connective tissue and in a variety of organs. They help connect many other types of cells together to form an organ.

Pygeum was found to be a potent inhibitor of rat prostatic fibroblast proliferation when these cells were exposed to growth factors that are normally present in prostate glands. The researchers theorize, "Our data suggest that the therapeutic effect of Pygeum africanum may be due at least in part to the inhibition of growth factors responsible for the prostatic overgrowth in man." They add, "We are not yet sure of the mechanism of action of Pygeum on cell proliferation but quite obviously it should not be mediated via the androgen delivery system of the cell, since Pygeum had no effect on 5-alpha-reductase activity or androgen receptor (unpublished results)."

As always with many of these herbal extracts, it will take quite a number of years before the full mechanisms of their actions are discovered.

The recommended dosage of Pygeum is 25 mg or 50 mg twice daily. Most of the pills on the market have between 25 mg and 100 mg or Pygeum extract. The majority will be standardized to contain about 13 percent of sterol extract. Therefore, a Pygeum pill that has 100 mg of the herbal extract will contain 13 mg of the active sterols.

Stinging Nettle (Urtica dioica) is a perennial herb with stinging hairs found in the United States mostly in forests, mountains, weedy, undisturbed areas and roadsides (Russel, 1997). Extracts of the roots have been used for the therapy of rheumatoid arthritis in Germany. One trademarked named in Europe is Bazoton. Extracts from Stinging nettle contain a number of substances including caffeic acid, malic acid (Obertries, 1996), polysaccharides (Wagner, 1989) and probably many other compounds, including lectins, lignans, and phytosterols.

The tolerability and effectiveness of a combination preparation comprised of SP and Urtica extract were tested in 2080 patients with mild to moderate prostate enlargement (Schneider, 1995). The study was done in the offices of hundreds of urologists in Germany. A before-and-after comparison revealed most patients showing an improvement in prostate symptoms and quality of life. For the most part, the treating doctors assessed the effectiveness of the preparation to be "good" or "very good." Out of the 2080 patients, only 15 were suspected to have developed mild side effects.

There has also been a study giving the combination of Urtica and Pygeum. The study was done in Warsaw, Poland and involved 134 patients (aged 53 to 84 years) who had symptoms of benign prostatic hyperplasia. The patients were randomly assigned to receive two capsules of the standard dose of an Urtica/Pygeum preparation (300 mg of Urtica dioica root extract combined with 25 mg of Pygeum bark extract) or two capsules containing half the standard dose twice daily for 8 weeks. After 28 days of treatment, urine flow increased and residual urine volume and nocturia were significantly reduced in both treatment groups. After 56 days of treatment, further significant improvements were noted in both groups. Only 5 out of the 134 patients reported any adverse effects and no one discontinued the treatment because of these side effects.

How does Urtica work? The mechanisms of this herb are not clearly understood. However, one possibility is that specific extracts of Urtica have the ability to influence a protein in blood, called serum hormone binding globulin (SHBG), to bind itself to prostate cells (Hryb, 1995). SHBG carries testosterone and estrogen with it in the bloodstream, and it also can go into the prostate gland. It's possible that this protein, by binding to prostate cells, influences their growth. By blocking this binding, Urtica could help prevent another way that the prostate gland can enlarge.

A further mechanism could be Urtica's ability to block inflammatory chemicals within the prostate tissue. One of these is leukotriene B4 (Obertries, 1996). With time scientists will find additional mechanisms by which extracts from Urtica influence prostate tissue.

Each of these herbs has a different method of action. As reviewed in a previous chapter, the growth of the prostate gland could have many causes. By addressing many of these factors, the response rate could be higher and patients would get more benefit than just taking one herb, or by just taking one drug, such as Proscar, that has one way of working, that is, blocking the conversion of testosterone to DHT.

The recommended dose of Urtica is 50 to 150 mg twice daily, although the research with this herb is more limited than with SP and more information is certainly required before giving any firm recommendations.

Rye Pollen Extract, known in Europe by the brand name Cernilton, has been used for the treatment of chronic prostatitis. Cernilton is an extract of rye pollen derived from several different plants in southern Sweden. It is rendered free of allergens and its two principle active constituents are a water-soluble fraction, T-60, and an acetone soluble fraction GBX (Buck, 1990). The acetone-soluble fraction has been found to consist of three beta-sterols with a similar chemical structure to stigmasterol (Kvanta, 1968). SP also contains a plant sterol called stigmasterol.

In 1990, researchers at the Department of Urology, University Hospital of Wales in Cardiff, gave two capsules of Cernilton twice a day to 60 patients with BPH. Each capsule of Cernilton contained 63 mg of pollen extract. The study was done in a double-blind, placebo-controlled manner and was conducted for a period of six months. Sixty-nine percent of the patients had improvement in their symptoms compared to 30 percent of those who received placebo pills. Patients on Cernilton had a significant decrease in the amount of urine in their bladder, and ultrasound examination showed a decrease in the size of the prostate. However, differences between placebo and the treated group were similar in terms of flow rate and the amount of urine voided. The researchers state, "It is concluded that Cernilton has a beneficial effect in BPH and may have a place in the treatment of patients with mild or moderate symptoms of outflow obstruction."

In 1991, Japanese researchers discovered that Cernilton was an effective medicine in the therapy of prostatitis (Suzuki, 1991). The patients noted no side effects. Prostatitis is an inflammation of the prostate gland. It can either be due to infectious causes, or it can be due to immune cells attacking certain prostate cells.

Two years later, a group from Germany gave Cernilton, in a dose of 1 tablet three times a day for 6 months for the treatment of chronic prostatitis to 90 patients (Rugendorff, 1993). At the conclusion of the study, 78 percent showed improvement, while 36 percent were cured of their symptoms.

In more recent study done in 1996, Japanese researchers showed rye pollen extract to have mild beneficial effects in up to 85 percent of patients with BPH (Yasumoto, 1995). The pollen extract was administered in a dosage of 126 mg three times a day for 12 weeks. This was confirmed by a Polish study (Dutkiewicz, 1996). A total of 51 patients with BPH were given Cernilton and compared to a group that received Tadenan (product name for Pygeum). Improvement was noted in 78 percent of the patients on Cernilton compared to only 55 percent of the Pygeum-treated patients.

What is it in rye pollen extract that leads to improvements in prostate symptoms? Scottish researchers have discovered a number of compounds within pollen, and at least one seems to have the ability to inhibit the growth of prostate cells (Habib, 1995). The chemical structure has been identified as a cyclic hydroxamic acid. This chemical has also been found to inhibit prostate cancer cell growth, too (Zhang, 1995).

As mentioned earlier, stigmasterol has also been found in pollen extract, so have the flavonoids quercitin and cernitin (Humiczewska, 1994). In the future, it's likely more compounds within this plant will be discovered.

Rye pollen extract is likely to gradually become more popular. This extract may be added to a number of products for prostate relief including products that already contain SP or Pygeum.

Epilobium: I have spent countless hours at the University of California Biomedical Library thumbing through dozens of journals regarding the latest research on herbs and plants. It is amazing how many new chemicals are constantly being discovered in these plants. Practically every issue of a journal relating to herbs mentions a new substance found in a plant that had previously been unknown. It will take many years, if not decades, before these chemicals are first tested in vitro in the lab, then tested in rodents, and then finally tried in humans.

One such herb is Epilobium. It is not yet well known in the US. I came across this herb by chance while thumbing through the journal *Planta Medica* (Ducrey, 1997). It caught my eye because the title of the article mentioned that extracts from this herb were able to inhibit the function of the enzyme 5-alpha-reductase, which converts testosterone to dihydrotestosterone (DHT).

There are a variety of species of Epilobium, and some of these have been used in folklore for a number of conditions including the treatment of bladder, kidney, and prostate disorders. They are even used in some parts of Russia as a tea. Epilobium is also known as Fireweed and as willow herb.

Epilobium, not unlike many plants, is rich in flavonoids. The particular ones within Epilobium are quercitin, isoquercitin, myricitrin, and isomyrcitrin. Other compounds include fatty acids, gallic, chlorogenic, and ellagic acids (Lesuisse, 1996). Recently, certain other substances have been extracted from Epilobium, which indicate it to have a possible role in the therapy of BPH. These two substances are in the family of ellagitannins and are named oenothein A and oenothein B (Lesuisse, 1995). Another flavonoid, called myricetin 3-O-beta-D-glucoronide, has been isolated and has been found to exhibit very strong anti-inflammatory abilities (ten times more than indomethacin, a nonsteroidal anti-inflammatory drug). This chemical also has an inhibitory effect on prostaglandin biosynthesis (Hiermann, 1991).

There have been no formal human studies published using Epilobium in the therapy of prostate enlargement, however, this herb looks promising. It has several compounds, especially oenothein B, which have been found in limited studies to block the conversion of testosterone to DHT (Lesuisse, 1995).

Oenothein B has also been reported to have antiviral and antitumor activities (Miyamoto, 1993).

At this point, though, since the research with this herb on humans is limited, it is difficult to predict how effective it will be. The appropriate dosage is also as yet uncertain.

Green tea: Certain compounds within green tea have structures similar to the ellagitannins found in Epilobium, and are also thought to inhibit 5-alpha-reductase (Liao, 1995).

Over the next few years science will discover dozens of different compounds within herbs that also block the 5-alpha-reductase enzyme. In the meantime, go ahead and have a glass or two of this green tea.

Beta-sitosterol: In 1995, a study was published in *Lancet,* the well-known British medical journal, evaluating the role of beta-sitosterol in the therapy of prostate enlargement (Berges, 1995). Beta-sitosterol is a plant-derived sterol, also known as a phytosterol. Although the active substance in this study was beta-sitosterol, the actual product used was called Harzol, trademarked by the German pharmaceutical company Hoyer GmbH & Co, headquartered in Neuss. Harzol is standardized to contain 10 mg of beta-sitosterol along with a mixture of phytosterols, including campesterol, and stigmasterol. SP contains a variety of phytosterols including beta-sitosterol, campesterol and stigmasterol. A number of other herbs are also known to contain these, and other, phytosterols.

In a randomized, double-blind, placebo-controlled study, 200 patients with symptoms of BPH were given two of these pills three times a day and were compared to a group that received a placebo. The study lasted 6 months and was done at the Department of

Urology and Biostatistics, Ruhr-University, in Bochum, Germany. Treatment with beta-sitosterol resulted in better urine flow and a decrease in residual urine in the bladder. There was no decrease in the size of the prostate gland. The researchers concluded, "Significant improvements in symptoms and urinary flow parameters show the effectiveness of beta-sitosterol in the treatment of benign prostatic hyperplasia." This study was sponsored by Hoyer.

Harzol has been tested in Europe since the early 1980s (Szutrely, 1982). Back in 1982, 23 patients had an ultrasound of their prostate gland before and after a two-month treatment with this medicine. Therapy with Harzol was effective in changing the echo structure of the prostate gland. The researchers interpreted this as a reduction in swelling within the prostate gland.

Beta-sitosterol has other interesting functions and effects on the human body. When human colon cancer cells were supplemented with beta-sitosterol, growth inhibition occurred (Awad, 1996). This is a good sign since uncontrolled growth is a marker for cancer formation. Long-term studies will need to be conducted on humans in order to know for sure how beta-sitosterol and other phytosterols influence a variety of tissues.

Beta-sitosterol is added to some SP products at a dose of 5 to 25 mg.

South African Star Grass: Also known by the genus name of Hypoxis rooperi, this plant is found mostly in southern Africa (Nicoletti, 1992). The extracts are taken from the roots of the plant and are marketed in Germany as Harzol, whereas in South Africa the dried corm material (fleshy, underground stem) is marketed as Prostamin for the treatment of prostate enlargement.

One of the primary compounds in this root is beta-sitosterol, which, as previously discussed, is found in a number of other plants. Glycosides and hypoxoside are other compounds isolated from Hypoxis.

The effective dosages and extracts for Hypoxis have not been evaluated as well as they have for SP. The clinical experience by U.S. doctors with this herb is very limited. Therefore, no definite guidelines about dosages can be given at this time. Whether extracts from Hypoxis are effective in treating BPH are currently not fully determined.

Pumpkin Seed (Cucurbita pepo): Sometimes a SP product will contain pumpkin seed extract. The seeds or extracts are currently used in Germany for the therapy of BPH (Dreikorn, 1995).

Back in 1994, researchers in China gave three oil extracts from pumpkin seeds to rabbits (Zhang, 1994). They observed that one of these extracts was able to reduce bladder pressure, increase bladder compliance, and reduce the pressure on the urethra. Formal, long-term human studies evaluating the role of pumpkin seed ingestion or extracts in relation to size of prostate gland have not been published.

Studies have been done using extracts of pumpkin seeds in combination with SP. The product name is Curbicin, and it is available in Europe. Curbicin contains 160 mg of extract PS6 from pumpkin seeds and also 80 mg of SP.

Drs. Carbin and Larsson, from the Department of Urology ant Karolinska Hospital in Stockholm, Sweden, performed a double-blind, placebo-controlled trial giving Curbicin to 53 patients for a period of 3 months. Urinary flow increased and, frequency and amount of urine left in the bladder improved from this therapy. We do know that SP helps patients with BPH. Whether pumpkin seed extracts had a role to play in the improvement of these patients is not known.

No recommendations can be made at this time whether the addition of pumpkin seeds or extracts of these seeds will benefit men with BPH. They certainly can't hurt. One study has shown that pumpkin seed oil is rich in antioxidants (Fahim, 1995). If a health care practitioner thinks a patient may benefit from compounds found in pumpkin seeds, all the patient has to do is ingest an ounce or so of these seeds a day (raw would be preferable) or take pumpkin seed extract in capsules. Some products marketed for prostate health contain pumpkin seed extract along with SP. I see no problem with this combination.

The oil content of pumpkin seeds is about 50 percent, and there are four predominant fatty acids within it: palmitic, stearic, oleic, and linoleic (Murkovic, 1996). These four make up 98 percent of the total oil content of the seed.

Zinc: This mineral is essential for normal growth and reproduction, tissue repair, and wound healing. It is also an essential component of a number of enzymes in the body. But what role does it play in the prostate gland?

It has been well established that, compared to other organs, the prostate gland accumulates extremely high levels of zinc (Liu, 1997). It is also known that much higher levels of zinc, and magnesium, are found in BPH than in regular-sized prostate glands (Dutkiewicz, 1995). Conversely, zinc levels are low in prostate cancer (Tvedt, 1989). However, despite considerable research over the past few years, the exact role of zinc in relation to the prostate gland has not been fully determined.

There have been numerous articles written in alternative magazines recommending the use of zinc in the therapy of BPH. Many of these were based on a 1993 study done with rodents (Fahim 1993). A group of rats was given an injection of 10 mg of zinc directly into their prostate gland, another group received 20 mg, while the third group received no zinc. Results showed significant reduction in prostate weight and activity of 5-alpha-reductase in the rats given the zinc. The higher dose zinc was more effective.

A review of the scientific literature does not indicate any extensive, formal studies done on the use of oral zinc in the therapy of human BPH. Studies in laboratories have not provided clear explanations. In a 1984 study, low amounts of zinc added to specimens of human prostate tissue increased the activity of 5-alpha-reductase, but at a higher concentration the activity of the enzyme was inhibited (Leake, 1984). The relevance of this study to actual human oral ingestion of zinc is difficult to predict. In 1988, Dr. A. Pinelli and colleagues, from the Department of Pharmacology at the University of Milan, in Italy, gave large doses of cimetidine (Tagamet, an anti-ulcer drug) for 45 days to rats. The levels of zinc in the prostate gland decreased while the weight of the prostate gland also decreased. The results of this study would indicate that lowering zinc levels decreases prostate size. The researchers state, "Since the zinc ion is essential to the prostate growth and androgen action and since cimetidine lowers prostate zinc content, the weight loss of the prostate observed in cimetidine treated animals can be reasonably attributed to the removal of zinc."

Therefore, whether one should incorporate zinc in the therapy of BPH, is, at this time, a difficult question to answer. As mentioned earlier in this section, enlarged prostate glands contain a very high amount of zinc. Many products with SP and Pygeum also have zinc added to them. Patients using these products benefit, but no one knows whether zinc had a role to play.

At this point, it would be better to focus on getting adequate amounts of some of the herbal extracts discussed above. There has been more evidence supporting their use as opposed to zinc. However, if a health care practitioner has recommended zinc, and the patient finds that it helps, by all means continue taking this mineral. If an herbal product contains reasonable amounts of this mineral, such as 5 to 15 mg, I wouldn't see a problem with using this product. Zinc could even be beneficial in terms of immune enhancement. Higher doses can lead to nausea. Excessive doses of zinc are not recommended for prolonged periods since copper deficiency may occur.

Plant Estrogens, Flavonoids, and Carotenoids: The use of plant estrogens or phytoestrogens was discussed in Chapter Five. Ingesting more and a wider variety of legumes, soy products, fruits and vegetables will ensure that you are getting the hundreds of beneficial plant chemicals. Some of these may have an enormous influence on the prostate gland.

There are also soy extracts that are being sold, such as genistein powder. No formal research is yet available regarding the use of this powder in terms of its effects on the prostate gland. However, it may theoretically hold promise. I would recommend, though, that whole foods, such as soy products, are not neglected and extracts taken only if there is a strong dislike for the taste of soy. Also, make sure to consume a variety of legumes. Incorporate in the diet lima, kidney, white, kudzu, pinto, and garbanzo beans, along with a number of different peas.

Melatonin: Nature's Prostate-Shrinking Sleeping Pill?
By now, most people have heard of the small gland in the brain, called the pineal gland, that releases the hormone melatonin at night that helps in falling and staying asleep. When young, the pineal gland is healthy and puts out an adequate amount of this hormone. As the body ages, the levels progressively decline. It is believed that the decline in the levels of melatonin with age contributes to the age-associated increase in the incidence of insomnia.

Over the past few years, scientists have learned that melatonin has an influence on a variety of tissues within the body. Receptors for melatonin have been found in heart tissue, spleen, colon, immune cells, and even the prostate gland. The fact that prostate gland cells have receptors on them has intrigued researchers. It is known that melatonin has an influence on seasonal reproduction and in development during puberty. It follows that it would have an influence on genitourinary tissues.

Drs. Eli Gilad and Nava Gisapel from the Department of Neurobiochemistry, George Wise Faculty of Life Sciences, and Dr. Haim Matzkin, from the Department of Urology, Tel Aviv Medical Center at Tel Aviv University in Israel, have been studying the role of melatonin in sleep for many years. They've also started to evaluate the role of melatonin in prostate tissue. In 1996, they announced that specific binding sites for melatonin were found on human prostate tissue (Laudon, 1996). Melatonin has also been shown to suppress human prostatic cell growth (Gilad, 1997) and is known to shrink reproductive areas including testicles, prostate, epididymis, and ovaries in rodents (Shirima, 1982; Sriuilai, 1989).

Although no formal studies have yet been published evaluating the role of melatonin in shrinking human prostate tissue, there is a possibility that this hormone may eventually be found to be helpful in the therapy of BPH. The dose necessary for this use is currently unknown. However, if a man with BPH, also has difficulty sleeping, it would certainly be worthwhile to try melatonin. I do not, at this time, recommend nightly use of this hormone since we don't know the long-term effects of continuous use. However, using it every other night, or two or three times a week seems appropriate. I have followed many patients on melatonin for over three years and no noteworthy side effects are reported when the dosages are kept low, such as 0.5 mg, and patients don't use this pill every night. I have personally taken melatonin twice a week for more than three years without side effects. In fact, my sleep is better now than it has ever been.

I don't see any problems with the use melatonin as part of a regimen that includes herbs or pharmaceutical medicines. The side effects to look out for with melatonin include vivid dreaming, grogginess in the morning, and tiredness. These are infrequent on dosages less than 0.5 mg.

As melatonin is for nighttime use, it wouldn't make sense for a vitamin company to add it to their SP formula.

Summary

BPH is caused by a number of factors that, together, cause the symptoms that annoy many older men. There are a variety of herbs and nutrients that play a role in the therapy of prostate enlargement. Some of these nutrients and herbs work by a different mechanism, therefore, it makes sense that the combination could theoretically have a synergistic effect. Chapter Fifteen discusses the practical ways of using these natural alternatives.

As to the choice between using drugs or herbs, one prominent Dutch researcher, Dr. J.L.H. Rudd Bosch, from the Department of Urology, Academic Hospital Rotterdam-Dijkzigt, in the Netherlands, gives his opinion. After reviewing the currently available published evidence, he concludes, "The results obtained with some of the phytotherapeutic drugs [herbs] are at least as good as the results obtained with finasteride and alpha-blockers."

With time, we will have better studies done for longer periods of time. These should give us a better idea on the role and effectiveness of the nutrients and herbs discussed in this chapter. We are also likely to discover other herbs or nutrients that could help reduce symptoms of BPH.

CHAPTER 10

Drugs and Cuts: Traditional Ways to Treat BPH

A visit to the family doctor, internist, or urologist, to complain of symptoms of prostate enlargement, will result in some questions and follow up with a physical exam to see if the prostate gland is swollen. The finger examination of the prostate gland will determine if the gland is enlarged uniformly or whether there's an area that happens to be harder than normal. A hard growth could indicate a tumor has developed while an even and smooth enlargement indicates that this is a simple case of BPH (benign prostate enlargement).

Assuming it is a simple case of BPH, and some form of therapy is requested, the doctor will pull out a prescription pad and write down the name of a drug and how often to take it. The pharmacy will fill out the prescription (hopefully covered by insurance) and taking the pills begins. Chances are there will be some relief.

There are a number of medicines that are prescribed to treat BPH. They generally fall into two categories. These include 5-alpha-reductase inhibitors and alpha-blockers. A discussion of the advantages and drawbacks of each of these types of drugs follows.

5-Alpha-reductase Inhibitors

The most commonly used 5-alpha-reductase inhibitor is Proscar (finasteride). Proscar is marketed as a selective inhibitor of 5-alpha-reductase, the enzyme that blocks the conversion of testosterone to dihydrotestosterone (DHT). DHT is one of the culprits in stimulating the growth of the prostate gland.

In some cases, finasteride lowers the DHT concentration in prostatic tissue by up to 85 percent (McConnell, 1992). It is prescribed at 5 mg once a day. Although Proscar is the most popular medicine used to treat prostate enlargement, a number of studies comparing it to placebo have shown mixed results. Some of these studies have shown the drug to have clear benefits, while others have shown no statistically significant improvement in the symptoms of patients (Eri, 1997). However, Proscar has shown clear benefits when studies have restricted its use to those who have very large prostates (Boyle, 1996). Although the fastest decrease in prostate size occurs in the first three months, it's possible the full benefits of Proscar may not be evident right away and could continue up to a year after initiation (Gormley, 1992; Lepor, 1996). Most doctors are now starting to recommend Proscar only for men who have very large prostate glands.

Proscar will not, by itself, be extremely effective. Prostate enlargement has many causes, not just the influence of DHT. Just blocking the conversion of testosterone to DHT is not going to solve the whole problem.

As a rule, the benefits of Proscar therapy are maintained as long as the medicine is continued (Monda, 1993). It is unclear whether the use of Proscar for many years will induce enough shrinkage to provide continued symptom relief after discontinuing the medicine. Most of the time Proscar is well tolerated by patients. Unfortunately, it does have an unpopular side effect: A small percentage of men lose their sex drive (Andersen, 1995).

Alpha-blockers

As the prostate gland enlarges, it causes pressure on the urethra, the outlet from which urine flows outward. There are certain muscle cells around the urethra, especially where it starts by the bladder. These muscle cells can sometimes constrict (increase in tone) and contribute to the narrowing of the urethral outlet. There are certain receptors on these muscle cells called alpha-receptors. When a medicine is ingested that stimulates these alpha-receptors, the muscle tightens and it becomes even more difficult to urinate. Certain amphetamine-like medicines, such as diet pills or cold medicines (pseudoephedrine), are a classic example: they make it difficult to urinate. On the other hand, there are drugs that block these receptors and these are often prescribed to patients who have difficulty urinating. These medicines are called alpha-blockers, and they generally provide improvement within two weeks after the initiation of therapy. Compare this to 5-alpha-reductase inhibitors that take much longer to reach their maximum effect (Eri, 1997).

Alpha-blockers were originally prescribed for the treatment of high blood pressure. There are tiny muscles around blood vessels that can contract and thus elevate blood pressure. Alpha-blockers work by relaxing these muscles and reduce blood pressure.

There are also tiny muscles present surrounding the urethra. Since alpha-blockers are also able to relax these muscles, they work quickly to improve symptoms. However, they are not curative. They don't lead to reversal of prostate enlargement since they don't attack the underlying problem. When alpha-blockers are stopped, prostate symptoms quickly return (Fabricius, 1990). However, if quick temporary relief from an annoying case of prostate enlargement is wanted, alpha-blockers are a good option. They can ease the symptoms until SP and other herbs are started. The herbal medicines will work slower, but in the meantime the number of times the patient must wake up at night to visit the bathroom is reduced.

The best known of the alpha-blockers are terazosin, prazosin, alfuzosin, and doxazosin. Side effects of alpha-blockers include dizziness, fatigue, a drop in blood pressure on standing, and weakness. These can occur in more than 20% of users (Eri, 1995). These medicines require caution, especially if the patient is currently on pills that lower blood pressure.

New alpha-blockers are constantly being introduced to the market. Tamsulosin (Flomax), an alpha-blocker for the therapy of BPH, received approval by the FDA in 1997. The recommended dosage is 0.4 mg once daily. Common side effects include dizziness and abnormal ejaculation.

In addition to the above, other medicines, hormones and nutrients may have the ability to inhibit the conversion of testosterone to DHT, or somehow shrink the prostate gland. These include spironolactone, bromocriptine, and others. These medicines are not commonly used since their full effects are currently not fully determined.

Alpha-blockers versus SP

In the limited studies done thus far comparing SP to alpha-blockers, SP has often, but not always, shown comparable benefits. When 41 men with BPH were randomized to receive SP or prazosin for 12 weeks, improvements in urinary frequency and urinary flow rate were slightly better for prazosin, but otherwise were very similar (Adriazola, 1992).

In one interesting study with 358 patients, alfuzosin, an alpha-blocker, was compared to Pygeum. The alpha-blocker worked a little bit better, but overall the symptom reduction in both groups was alike (Abbou, 1996). In another study, alfuzosin was compared to SP (Grasso, 1995). Sixty-three patients with BPH were tested in a double-blind manner for a three-week period using alfuzosin 2.5 mg three times a day compared to SP 160 mg twice a day. There were clear differences between the two treatments. The group on alfuzosin showed statistically significant improvement in the ability to urinate, and had a better peak flow rate (the speed of the urine coming out of the bladder). The results of this study make sense since alpha-blockers are known to act very quickly and the effects of SP would take longer to notice. In the short term, alpha-blockers, as a rule, are probably more effective than single herbs. However, the combination of two or more herbs working with a different mechanism could, in the long run, potentially be more beneficial than alpha-blockers used alone. More research is needed to evaluate this proposal.

Surgery

There are times when your prostate gland may be extremely enlarged and surgery could be a viable option.

The primary method of treating a severely enlarged prostate gland is by a surgical procedure known as transurethral resection of the prostate, or by its acronym TURP. It is accepted that, in severe cases, surgery produces a far greater improvement than drugs (Guess, 1995). There are drawbacks, though. The expense of surgery, the possibility that something could go wrong during the operation or anesthesia, lost time from work, and pain. In a study done in the 1980s on more than 3800 patients who underwent TURP, at least 25% of the patients had some kind of surgical complication (Mebust, 1989). Furthermore, at least 2 people out of a thousand died within 30 days of the surgery. Some of the complications associated with surgery include incontinence and impotence.

Laser surgery is an alternative to TURP. A laser is introduced through the urethra and up to the prostate area. Any excessive prostate tissue causing blockage can be destroyed. This procedure is relatively new and it will take time for urologists to fine-tune their skills.

But can surgery be avoided? More and more users of SP are finding out that this herb can either prevent the need for surgery, or at least postpone its need. Jim L., an investment advisor who lives in Los Angeles, is one example. He says:

I'm a 47 year-old male who began to experience symptoms of an enlarged prostate about six years ago. The typical sensations and accom-

panying behaviors emerged as a set of undesirable changes in my life. Until about 6 months
ago, I was getting up each night to urinate from
1 to 3 times. I naturally reacted to such inconven-
iences by trying to curtail my liquid intake,
which brought on other symptoms; notably
those associated with mild dehydration. My wife
complained that my getting up at night was
interrupting her sleep. Other symptoms relating
to sexual performance were disturbing as well.

I felt uncomfortable most of the time, including those moments before and after urination.
The sensation I felt in my lower urinary area
was like having a tennis ball pushing against my
urinary tract.

When I brought up these symptoms with my
doctor, he referred me to a specialist who recommended surgery. Descriptions of exploratory
surgery were so repulsive that I never returned
for a second appointment.

Quite by accident, I learned about SP, and
since early December 1996, I've been taking
minimal doses, in addition to Pygeum extract.
I feel pleased to report that, without any other
changes in my diet or behavior patterns, my
symptoms are nearly completely gone. I regularly sleep without interruption and have no
discomfort with urination. Urine flow has significantly increased (although not as strong as
my 14 year-old son's has). These changes are
occurring with one additional interesting effect:
I've noticed that, in the past couple of months
(after 3 months of use), I have not been experiencing any hair loss.

Summary

Alpha-blockers and 5-alpha-reductase inhibitors are certainly helpful in the therapy of prostate enlargement. Alpha-blockers generally work quicker than herbal products and they may be appropriate to use temporarily if symptoms are very uncomfortable.

It's quite likely that therapy with medicines will delay the need for surgery. But can these medicines completely prevent the eventual need for the scalpel? It's too soon to tell.

CHAPTER 11

SP and Prostate Cancer

Prostate cancer is the most common non-skin malignancy in the United States with an occurrence of about 250,000 new cases a year. The majority of these cancers are localized, meaning they are present within the prostate gland and have not spread outside. It is estimated that the incidence could rise to 330,000 cases over the next few years, with more than 40,000 deaths predicted for the year 1997 (Wingo, 1995).

Long-term human studies evaluating SP and its role in cancer have not been done. One of the few clues we have about the influence of some of the compounds found within SP on tumor cells come from a 1997 study done at Purdue University in West Lafayette, Indiana. Drs. Hiroko Shimada, Varro Tyler, and Jerry McLaughlin isolated two compounds from SP berries, called mono-laurin and mono-myristin. These compounds showed moderate activity against certain kidney and pancreatic cancer cells, and borderline activity against certain prostatic cancer cells. (Shimada, 1997)

The clinical significance of these findings is currently unclear. However, Dr. McLauglin has some thoughts. He says, "As far as we know, there are no carcinogenic compounds in SP that we know of. Moreover, there is a potential for anti-tumor substances within SP. Theoretically, there is a possibility that SP may protect against cancer but unless actual human studies are done, we're not going to know for sure. There are countless compounds within nature that have anti-tumor activities. The National Cancer Institute has shown some interest in examining many old compounds and molecules in nature that may have good applications. For instance, one of my scientific colleagues has found that betulinic acid, from birch trees, knocks out melanoma cells."

In 1996, Ravenna and colleagues, from the Department of Experimental Medicine and Pathology, University of La Sapienza, in Rome, determined in laboratory studies that extracts of SP have some inhibitory activity against a certain hormone-dependent prostate cancer. However, it is extremely premature to extrapolate the results from a lab study done with isolated cells to a full human being.

Can Reducing DHT Levels Influence Prostate Cancer?

One of the concerns I often hear from users of medicines that influence DHT levels is whether this could somewhat influence, in a positive or negative way, the growth of prostate cancer. Although the full evidence is not yet in, at least one new study shows that cancerous cells in prostate tissue have many times higher levels of 5-alpha-reductase enzyme than noncancerous prostate cells (Bjelfman, 1997).

Does this mean that taking Proscar or SP, or any medicine that blocks the conversion of testosterone to DHT, or blocks the action of DHT, would reduce the risk of prostate cancer? This is a theoretical possibility, but until actual studies are done, it will not be known for certain.

Conventional Treatment of Prostate Cancer

Depending on the severity of the cancer, there are a few options available. Since many prostate cancers are small, are localized to the prostate gland, and grow very slowly, the wait-and-see approach is quite reasonable. A man is often more likely to die from another medical cause before the prostate cancer has a chance to grow, spread, and cause difficulties. If a patient and his doctor decide to wait and observe, routine prostate exams need to be performed. The blood test, PSA (prostate specific antigen), should be done regularly to see if the levels are increasing. PSA levels in the blood can indicate the severity of the cancer. If the levels rise, this means it is more likely that the cancer is growing.

Other options to cancer therapy include surgery, radiation therapy, freezing, and hormone therapy. For more detailed information, consult a urologist, or purchase a book on this topic.

Does SP Influence PSA?

One of the ways doctors monitor patients with prostate enlargement, or patients with a suspicious growth in the prostate gland is to do a blood test known as PSA (prostate specific antigen). As a rule, the higher the PSA level, the more likelihood of an existing cancer within the prostate gland. However, therapy with Proscar (finasteride) is known to reduce PSA levels, making it more difficult to monitor any existing or developing prostate cancer. Could therapy with SP also reduce PSA levels?

This matter has not been determined yet. It is not known for certain at this time whether giving someone SP or other herbs will influence the amount of PSA released into the bloodstream. It is known, though, that finasteride will generally reduce PSA levels by about 50 percent. A group of researchers who participated in the finasteride study group financially supported by Merck & Co report that for an individual on finasteride, one can get an approximate value of the true value of a patient's PSA test by doubling their PSA level (Oesterling, 1997).

Summary

Preliminary laboratory studies using cell cultures indicate that there may be compounds within SP that have some anti-tumor activity. Whether SP administration to humans will have a role in cancer prevention or therapy is currently undetermined.

As a last note, I need to mention that a review of all the studies determining the role of exercise in the incidence of prostate cancer has not found a clear connection (Oliveria, 1997).

CHAPTER 12

Skin and Hair

Hormones, especially testosterone, are definitely involved in the health of hair and skin. Testosterone is found in practically every type of tissue including hair, skin and breast. As discussed in Chapter Seven, testosterone is converted in skin and hair into dihydrotestosterone (DHT), a more potent hormone. An excess of DHT production is linked to a variety of skin disorders such as acne, and even male pattern baldness. An excess amount of DHT interrupts the hair-growth cycle on the scalp by gradually shrinking hair follicles. A condition known as idiopathic female hirsutism (basically, excess hair in the wrong places) is also believed to be due to an overproduction of DHT.

As mentioned earlier, SP is known not only to go to prostate tissue, but to also find its way to skin. In fact, a study in 1984 did show that extracts from SP were able to inhibit androgen metabolism and binding in human foreskin fibroblasts (Sultan, 1984). Fibroblasts are special cells found in skin, specifically connective tissue, that help make collagen. It is likely that SP could have an influence on a variety of skin cells, including sebaceous glands, those little glands that can grow into annoying big pimples. I, personally, have had occasional pimples ever since my teenage years. Although in the past few years the problem has been minimal, I noticed that hardly any pimples developed since I began taking SP. I'm only 40 and don't have prostate problems, but I was taking it while writing this book. I wanted to see if it had any side effects and how it would influence my hair and skin. Also, some reddish areas of my face have turned a healthier skin tone. As to the influence of SP on hair, it is too early to tell. Hair loss takes several months, sometimes years to manifest itself. It is too soon to know what kind of influence SP has on hair loss.

Donald Brown, N.D., a specialist in herbal medicine from Seattle, Washington, thinks SP may play a role in skin, "I have used SP clinically with male and female acne patients with some help," he says, "Tea tree oil applied topically works well, too. I use a concentration of 5 to 15 percent."

Lise Alschuler, N.D., Chair of the Botanical Medicine Department at Bastyr University in Seattle, Washington, reports, "I've prescribed SP for cystic acne. Since I use a variety of naturopathic remedies, it's difficult to say whether SP had a major role to play in the improvement. I don't think the effects of SP have been remarkable, although patients report that it helps. Perhaps acne requires a much higher dose than 160 mg twice a day. I'm still experimenting."

What about SP's influence on oily skin? Anecdotal reports point to some benefits. One patient tells me, "I've been taking saw palmetto in combination with Pygeum africanum twice a day. I don't know if it does a thing for my hair but it has cleared up a perennial problem with oily skin.

Do Monkeys Need Toupees?

Just like humans, monkeys do get bald, too. In fact, stumptail monkeys have been found to lose their frontal hair in a manner similar to humans. The DHT level in the skin of their frontal scalp is very high. The activity of 5-alpha reductase, the enzyme that converts testosterone to DHT, is also very high in the frontal scalp of humans.

Herbal Hair-Raiser?

Thus far, I have mentioned that the conversion of testosterone to DHT occurs by an enzyme known as 5-alpha reductase. Now it's time to explain this matter in more detail. There are two types of enzymes that convert testosterone to DHT: 5-alpha reductase type 1 and 5-alpha reductase type 2. The 5-alpha reductase type 2 enzyme is found more prominently in prostate tissue, and also in other parts of the genitourinary system such as the epididymis and seminal vesicles (Silver, 1994; Jenkins, 1992). The 5-alpha reductase type 1 enzyme is found more prominently in skin and liver (Andersson, 1991). Proscar (finasteride) predominantly inhibits mostly the type 2 enzyme, while extracts from SP are reported in one study to inhibit both (Lehle, 1995). However, the claim of SP blocking the conversion of testosterone to DHT has not yet been proven. There is conflicting information on this matter. There is more convincing evidence, though, that SP may inhibit the action of DHT.

Even though finasteride (Proscar) is thought to primarily inhibit the type 2 enzyme, a study has shown that it can grow hair in men *(Modern Medicine,* 1997). Researchers at the University of California in San Francisco participated in an international, multicenter, randomized, placebo-controlled, double-blind study of more than 1,500 men younger than 45 who had mild to moderate male-pattern baldness. Half of the men took 1 mg a day of finasteride, while the other half took a placebo. When finasteride is given to patients with BPH, the usual dosage is 5 mg.

At the end of the study, photographs were taken of the men, and roughly half of them on the medicine showed significant hair growth compared to only 7% of those who took the placebo. The other half of the men on finasteride did not show any continued loss of hair.

One concludes from these results, that finasteride will probably become more popular. What's needed now is an evaluation of SP in hair growth. Could SP, since it has some androgenic blockade in the prostate gland, offer a similar promise in blocking androgens in scalp?

We don't know, but there are some individuals who think they have noticed results. The following reports were posted on the internet in the newsgroup alt.baldspot:

I take 320 mg a day, of the standardized saw palmetto and have had great results. A year ago I tried minoxidil alone with no results and now using minoxidil along with saw palmetto it is coming in great. My hairline has moved forward a bit and the spot on top is filled in nicely. There's more to go.

When I started taking SP almost 4 months ago, I was taking pure SP extract with no additions like Pygeum or pumpkin seeds or any of that stuff; and I was taking over 2,000 mg per day (four 585 mg capsules). After I noticed that it started working for me (in about a month), I began experimenting with combination supplements that contained both Pygeum and SP, and I also decreased the dosage a little to under 1,000 mg a day, thinking that the combos should be more potent. The recommended dose for prostate patients is around 300 mg so I figured that 2,000 mg was a bit excessive. After being on combos for 3 or 4 weeks, my hair started to get really weak again, like before I started the treatment. I couldn't brush it right and I started shedding normally again (the way I had before I had taken anything). This worried me, so I went back and got the same brand of SP extract that I had started with (585 mg) and returned to my original dosage. Within 2 weeks I could brush my hair normally again and after 3 weeks the shedding stopped.

Other reports posted indicated no benefit from SP in terms of hair growth.

Summary

The exact mechanism of how SP works is not known, therefore, it's difficult to say for sure how, or whether, this herb could help with skin and hair. If it were true that SP blocks the formation of DHT, or blocks the action of DHT, then it would make it more likely to influence the course of acne and hair loss.

It would be worthwhile for acne sufferers to explore the use of SP or some of the other herbs mentioned in this book. It's also worthwhile to try SP and other herbs for hair loss, especially if a prostate problem is being treated. We definitely need more research in the area of herbal influence on hair and skin.

CHAPTER 13

Interviews with Doctors and Researchers

There are countless natural nutrients and herbs that have an influence on health. Science has not yet fully evaluated all of these supplements. However, since many of these are available to the consumer, a number of people take them, and doctors use these supplements in their practice. Much anecdotal experience has accumulated.

Science generally frowns on anecdotes, and for good reason. They can sometimes be misleading, or inaccurate. However, sometimes clues can be gotten on how a medicine works in real life on real patients through anecdotes that can't be readily obtained through formal studies. Interesting effects of medicines can also be discovered from the actual users or doctors who are prescribing them. And that's the purpose of this chapter.

I interviewed a number of health care practitioners and individuals who have a great deal of experience with herbs. These interviews are presented in alphabetical order.

Lise Alschuler, N.D., is Chair of the Botanical Medicine Department at Bastyr University in Seattle, Washington. She regularly uses botanical medicines in her clinical practice.

"I use SP as my first choice, in a dose of 160 mg twice a day. If there's no improvement, I either change to a tea form of SP or the tincture. A few people don't respond to the capsules but they respond to the tea. Historically, saw palmetto tea has been used as a pelvic tonic because it may relax smooth muscles in the pelvis. I've also been known to prescribe SP at a dose of 160 mg four times a day. Occasionally someone may respond to this higher dose better than the lower dose. Once they respond to the higher dose, I'll gradually lower it to the level that keeps a patient satisfied.

"If the response to SP has not been adequate, I'll add Pygeum at a dose of 50 to 100 twice a day. I have not had patients report side effects on SP or Pygeum.

"If there's still no response to these two herbs, I prescribe Stinging nettle in the form of a tea. I've noticed that some people improve when Stinging nettle is added. This herb is sold in bulk form and it's easy to make tea from it. It's also available in capsules but I'm not aware that it's currently available in extract form.

"My regimen also includes zinc and pumpkin seeds, however, I think that their role is minor compared to the herbs."

James Balch, M.D., is a urologist in Trophy Club, Texas.

"In my experience, SP works about 50% of the time to improve symptoms of BPH. If SP, by itself, is not enough, then I add Pygeum to the therapy. This often brings the response rate up to 75%, and many patients are able to avoid surgery. I have not found any side effects with herbal therapies for BPH. If a patient does not respond to SP and Pygeum, I add finasteride (Proscar). Some patients respond very well to the combination of herbs and pharmaceutical medicines."

Stan Bazilian, M.D., is a physician in Philadelphia, Pennsylvania.

"I have a few patients on SP. All of them are not getting up at night as much as they used to. It usually takes about 2 weeks for the SP to be effective. No side effects have been reported."

Marie Bochniak, D.C., is Assistant Clinical Professor at Los Angeles College of Chiropractic.

"I have found saw palmetto to be useful in long-distance bicyclists. Sitting for hours or days on a bike can sometimes irritate and inflame their prostate gland. Many users of SP find relief of their prostate symptoms."

Cherry Briskey, N.D., is clinical faculty professor at South West Naturopathic Medical Center in Tempe, Arizona.

"I've had very good response to SP. Most of the men report a decrease in symptoms. Recently we've started treating a patient with polycystic ovary syndrome with SP in order to see if this herb can block some of the androgenic effects."

Donald Brown, N.D., is the author of *Herbal Prescriptions for Better Health,* (Prima, 1996), and President of Natural Product Research Consultants in Seattle, Washington.

"My top choice for treating BPH is SP, followed by beta-sitosterol. Other good options include Pygeum and nettles. I'm not a fan of pollen, although it could work well for chronic prostatitis. In my opinion, I don't think there's enough proof that zinc works.

"As to pumpkin seeds, the liposterolic extracts are approved to treat BPH in Germany. I think, though, that there's a lot of overlap between the actions of the different herbs that are high in fatty acids. They may have a similar method of interacting with prostate tissue.

"I personally don't have any objections to using finasteride with saw palmetto. I also don't have any problems using an alpha-blocker if necessary.

"Patients should realize that therapy for BPH might have to continue for a lifetime. If you stop using it, your symptoms could come back. I had a patient who flew to France on vacation and a few days later called me in a state of panic. He had forgotten his bottle at home, and now his symptoms had come back. He wanted to know if there were any stores in France where he could purchase this herb.

"The longest I've had a person on SP is 4 years and there's been no side effects reported."

Jim Duke, formally with the United States Department of Agriculture, has been a herbalist for many yeas, and is the author of *The Green Pharmacy* (Rodale Press, 1997). At age 68, Mr. Duke has prostate enlargement and takes a combination of various herbs.

"I like ingesting herbs as part of my diet and like to consume the whole herb as opposed to taking extracts, but I have no problems with people ingesting extracts. I eat pumpkin seeds for their zinc content, and brazil nuts since they have a high amount of selenium. Recently I learned that pinto beans have more genistein [an anti-cancer nutrient] than soybeans, so I've started eating more of them. I recently was involved in a research project and we analyzed 75 different legumes. Kudzu was found to have one of the highest amounts of genistein.

"As to the therapy of prostate enlargement, I prefer the shotgun approach. That is, using many different herbs at one time to help a person improve quicker. Most patients with BPH are too impatient to try one herb at a time. Using multiple herbs at one time could provide quicker relief.

"I have heard suggestions that SP may help in slowing down male pattern baldness, but I'm not aware of any studies that prove this."

Terry Grossman, M.D., is in private practice in Lakewood, California.

"The response of my patients to SP has been variable. Some report increased urine flow and a decrease in nocturia. I would say 40 to 50 percent notice an improvement. However, when I add Pygeum, the response usually increases to about 60 to 70 percent.

"I also give SP to male patients who are on DHEA. By the way, I used to prescribe high doses of DHEA in the past, but now I'm realizing that lower doses are effective with fewer side effects. I rarely use dosages more than 15 mg.

"Interestingly, I've had some luck treating BPH recently with a homeopathic medicine called Lycotodium. I'm not sure how it works."

Michael Janson, M.D., is President of the American College for the Advancement of Medicine and the author of *The Vitamin Revolution in Health Care.*

"Saw palmetto is unbelievable. I get very consistent results. Older men say their frequency at night drops from 3 or 4 to one. Recently I've started using it in combination with Pygeum and nettles."

Skye Lininger, D.C., in Portland, Oregon, reports treating more than 100 patients with SP.

"As a rule, at least 8 out of 10 patients respond to a combination of SP and Pygeum. I also use zinc and flax seed oil. Nettles is another herb I have been considering lately."

Bob Martin, D.C., is a chiropractic physician who also hosts a radio show on KFYI-AM 910, in Phoenix, Arizona.

"Saw palmetto is one of my top 10 favorite nutritional supplements—it's a home run for many patients. The longest I've treated an individual is 10 years, and there have been no side effects. Many times a patient happens to be on multiple medicines and nutrients and I try to minimize the number of medicines they are on by gradually eliminating each one. However, I can't do it with this herb. I have patients tell me, 'You're not taking my SP away from me.'

"SP works in most cases, but not all the time. If somebody is too far-gone, that is, their prostate gland is too large and their symptoms severe, they have to initially be medicated by a pharmaceutical drug for a period of time. However, they often get side effects, such as a lowering of sex drive, and they want to start SP as soon as possible.

"When SP is not completely effective, I add Pygeum. The combination is better than each one alone."

Jan McBarron, M.D., is board certified in Preventive Medicine and practices in Columbus, Georgia.

"SP is an herb with great medical value. I have one patient who has been on it for at least 8 years without any side effects. In my opinion, since enlargement of the prostate begins in men in their late 30s,

I think any man over age 40 should consider taking SP, perhaps a dose of 160 mg daily."

Rob McCaleb is President and Founder of Herb Research Foundation in Boulder, Colorado. I asked him about saw palmetto tea compared to the lipid extracts sold as capsules.

"Let's keep in mind that many fat-soluble compounds do make it in liquids. For instance, many aromatic oils in teas find themselves in the water. I would suspect, though, with our current extraction techniques, that the capsules sold in vitamin stores would have more active ingredients than just drinking the tea."

J. Jeffrey Mullahey, Ph.D., is Associate Professor at the Wildlife Ecology and Conservation at the University of Florida in Immokalee. He has extensive experience in the growth and harvesting of SP in Florida, and conducts various field studies. I asked him about the different botanical names that saw palmetto has been identified in the medical literature, and whether he thought products from different companies would be much different in their content of active ingredients.

"*Serenoa repens* is the correct botanical name, but *Sabal serulata* is sometimes used as the official name of saw palmetto. I think in the research papers they are referring to the same thing. Sometimes the older literature citation doesn't change, or some researchers in foreign countries may use *Sabal* instead of *Serenoa*.

"I suspect the contents of various products from different companies should be similar. Although the extraction process, such as the amount of heat used, could alter the final fatty acid content. Also, the soil where SP is grown could perhaps make a slight difference. The soil of Georgia is different from the soil in Florida. Whether this is going to alter the fatty acid content to any significant degree is difficult to tell.

"Florida recently established SP as an agricultural crop. This is different from its previous status. Before, if a person harvested somebody else's SP plants, they would be charged with a misdemeanor. Now, since the status of SP has changed to being an agricultural crop, it's a felony to harvest SP from someone else's land. You have to prove where you harvested the SP. There's always been a problem with people trespassing properties to harvest SP. Years ago, when there was little awareness about SP, landowners didn't care, or didn't pay attention to it. They can now make a very good supplemental income from SP; it can be a significant source of money. In Florida we currently have 5 major buyers, and a host of harvesters.

"At the present time we're conducting a study to answer the question whether there will be a shortage of plants as the demand increases. With the growing public awareness about SP, there's bound to be ever increasing need for more crop harvesting. However, SP is so widespread in South Eastern states that I doubt there will be a shortage. Farmers don't plant it; it's just there, growing naturally. Right now only a small portion of the state crop of Florida is harvested. As far as I know, SP is not grown in Europe and the Europeans will have to buy it from the States. There seems to be no better growing condition than in south Florida.

"We are concerned that the increasing harvesting of SP may not be good for the wildlife that relies on it as a source of food or shelter. These include raccoons, deer, hogs, and bears. SP is prime food for bear in the month of August.

"We get a fair number of contacts through our web site from men who have used SP. They give testimonials that it works. I've heard about the claims of increasing libido but no one I know has told me that it definitely works for sex improvement. I have talked to many men who told me incredible stories on how SP has helped them with their prostate enlargement. The medical community is behind the knowledge curve on SP, just like they are on many herbal remedies."

Richard Podell, M.D., is Clinical Professor, Department of Family Medicine at UMDMJ-Robert Wood Johnson Medical School in New Brunswick, New Jersey. He is board-certified in Internal Medicine and Family Medicine.

"The last five years has seen a remarkable growth in the number of double-blind research studies in the field of nutrition. These have validated many of the concepts that certain nutritional supplements are beneficial to human health. The stigma of doing research in nutrition has disappeared, and researchers are now more comfortable in focusing their efforts on finding the healing benefits of garlic, fish oils, vitamins, and so on.

"I practice scientific medicine with a holistic perspective. I started incorporating natural remedies in my practice a few years ago. I have used SP for 5 years now, most often combining it with Pygeum. Frankly, Proscar has been disappointing. Most urologists I talk to find it mediocre. For quick action on the prostate, I prefer Hytrin.

"In my practice, I would say more than 50% of patients on SP and Pygeum have improved. Although, I have to say that when it comes to treating BPH, studies show that the placebo effect is very high in treating this condition. The outflow of urine varies with stress, other medicines, possibly fat intake, and other factors. BPH has a variable course in people over time.

"Therefore, we have to be careful how we interpret the research findings, and the anecdotal experience of users. I would, though, say that I find the herbs are at least as effective as Proscar, and would choose the herbs over this medicine.

"Sometimes, if I have a patient who wants quick relief, I use the combination of Hytrin and the herbs. Hytrin, by relaxing the smooth muscle around the bladder outlet, will provide relief within days and gives the herbs the time to gradually start working. The disadvantage with Hytrin is that it does not treat the underlying problem.

"In addition to herbs, I remind my patients to eat less fat since at least one study has indicated that a high fat diet may stimulate not only prostate cancer, but also its enlargement."

Ascanio Polimeni, M.D., has a private practice in Milan and Rome.

"In Italy, many doctors commonly use SP 160 mg twice a day for prostate enlargement. The brand most commonly used is Permixon. In my practice I also use Pygeum 25 mg twice a day. I've recently started experimenting with giving SP to patients on DHEA and also recommending soy extracts such as genistein powder, one or two tablespoons a day mixed in water or fruit juice."

The Word from Health Food Stores

Suma Nathan is a nutritionist at Better Bodies Nutrition store in Las Vegas, Nevada

"SP is very popular these days. From the response of my clients, I would estimate that at least 60% are helped from the combination of SP and Pygeum. Other herbs that customers used for urinary tract problems include juniper berry, parsley extract and botchu."

David Stouder is the manager at Apple Health Foods in Redwood City, California

"I would say about 70% of my customers report improvement in their prostate symptoms from taking SP and other herbs."

CHAPTER 14

Frequently Asked Questions

Can I Take SP with Other Vitamins, Minerals and Herbs?

Anecdotal evidence from physicians who use SP and other herbs for the therapy of prostate symptoms doesn't indicate that these herbs present any problems when used in combination with other medicines or nutrients. However, formal studies have not been published regarding this issue.

Will Taking SP Prevent Some of the Side Effects from DHEA?

One of the theoretical problems in taking DHEA is the possibility that this hormone's conversion into testosterone, dihydrotestosterone (DHT), and estrogens, could potentially stimulate prostatic growth. Although there's no formal proof that this occurs, individual anecdotes have pointed to this possibility, especially with high doses of DHEA such as 15 mg or more. Most people consider 15 mg a low dose, however, I personally think the majority of users of these over the counter hormones are overdosing.

DHEA could accumulate in body tissues, and using it daily could eventually lead to side effects.

Is it possible that combining SP with DHEA or testosterone could reduce the possibility of unpleasant androgenic effects?

We don't have any human studies to indicate what the combination of DHEA or testosterone with SP will do. However, a French study done on rodents gives us some clues (Paubert-Braquet, 1996). In this trial, two groups of rats were chosen: 1) The first group was castrated and treated with estradiol and testosterone. 2) The second group was castrated, treated with estradiol and testosterone, but, in addition, was given SP.

After three months of continuous treatment with estradiol and testosterone, the first group had markedly increased prostate weight. The weight of the prostate gland in the second group, the ones also given SP did not change. The researchers stated, "These results demonstrate that administering LSESR (lipidosterolic extract of *Serenoa repens*, or SP) to hormone-treated castrated rats inhibits the increase in prostate wet weight. This effect of LSESR may explain the beneficial effect of this extract in human benign prostatic hypertrophy."

At this point it is unclear whether the human prostate gland would respond similarly to the rat prostate. However, for the time being, it would make sense for any man on DHEA or testosterone to also consider taking SP if clinical evaluation by a physician shows the hormone therapy is influencing the size of the gland.

As to whether a woman on DHEA would benefit from SP is currently not known. It may be worthwhile for clinicians to try the combination to see if SP prevents or decreases any of the side effects associated with DHEA, such as pimples and facial hair growth. However, if a woman is getting masculinizing effects from DHEA, her dose should be reduced.

How Do I Know the Products I Buy Over the Counter Actually Contain Active Ingredients?

You don't know for sure, unless you have the products tested yourself in a laboratory. However, the majority of products from well-known vitamin companies should be perfectly okay. In January of 1997, our center tested different DHEA products on the market and found them to be true to their label. The results were published in our January, 1997 newsletter (see the back of the book on how to order) and also posted on our web site at www.raysahelian.com.

Because of the wide interest in natural therapies, most of the vitamin companies are getting to be very large corporations grossing millions of dollars a year. They now have name brand recognition to uphold.

Will SP Increase My Sex Drive?

This is difficult to say. During formal studies done with SP, there have been rare mentions of individuals having an increased sexual drive. Searching the Internet revealed a few anecdotes posted from people who thought SP helped them.

I've been only using oral SP for a few months but I've not noticed much affect on my hair yet. I did notice an increase in libido.

* * *

I've noticed increased libido when taking 320 mg twice a day. The effect, though, is subtle.

As a pharmacist, I frequently compound SP with Pygeum. I use it mostly for patients with BPH, but bodybuilders use the formula, too, if they're taking androgenic steroids. Users do report an increase in sex drive.

Until formal, double-blind studies are done testing for SP's effect on libido, it's hard to give a definite answer at this time.

Is it Necessary to Pack SP Pills when Traveling?

Don't leave home without it. There's no guarantee that the country you're visiting will carry SP in their pharmacy or vitamin store. I've heard a few stories of men who became acquainted with bathrooms in foreign countries more frequently than they originally planned. Ed, a gentleman from Sherman Oaks, California, is one example. He relates, "I went on a trip to Europe and didn't take SP for 5 days. My symptoms of BPH came back and I was going to the bathroom at least half a dozen times at night. After I came back home, I resumed taking SP, and my symptoms improved promptly."

Does Everyone Benefit from SP?

No. The response rate is usually 40 to 80 percent. The addition of other herbs and nutrients raises this percentage higher. Some users don't get better, but find their symptoms are not progressively getting worse. Richard, a 70-year-old gentleman, tells me, "I've had symptoms of BPH for 9 years and never had a TURP. I think my BPH started after a bout of prostatitis. I went to my urologist and had a biopsy of the prostate along with a pyelogram (to check the kidneys and bladder), and other tests. My urologist told me there was no cancer. Over the years the symptoms continued. I would get up at night many times. With time, the symptoms progressed.

"I took Proscar for one year at a dose of 5 mg a day, but I didn't think it helped. I've been taking SP now at 160 mg twice a daily for close to a year. There's been no major change, but my symptoms are not getting worse. I haven't noticed any side effects. I'm still going to the bathroom three times at night."

Do the Benefits from SP Continue Forever?

The answer to this question is not clearly known, since the longest human study published with SP has been three years. Anecdotal responses from users indicate that a good number continue to benefit from long term use. However, in some individuals, the disease can progress with time. Sal relates this story. "I'm 63 years old. I had a vasectomy in 1972. My problem with BPH started in 1990 when I found myself making repeated trips to the bathroom at night. My PSA was normal and I was told that the prostate was not enlarged enough for surgery. At that time I started taking SP and other herbs and enjoyed immediate relief.

"Over the years I continued with the herbs using

various brands and combinations of ingredients with good results. However, the past year has been a different story. I find myself getting up 5–6 times a night, and checking every rest room on the interstate. The herbs no longer seem to work. I was just examined at a major clinic and was told I had no cancer, just an enlargement. They recommended I have surgery. In the meantime they gave me Hytrin saying it would give me some relief. The problem is that I normally have low blood pressure and the last thing I need to have is something that will make it lower.

"I'm not really interested in any of the normal surgery techniques for the prostate because the problem just seems to come back or the surgery generates additional problems. My brother-in-law has had surgery twice and my guess is he will be soon due for the third time."

Is SP Useful for Prostatitis?

Anytime the suffix 'itis' added to a medical term, it means there's some type of inflammation going on. Prostatitis means the prostate gland is inflamed, but it doesn't specify the cause of inflammation. There are two major categories of prostatitis: infectious, and non-infectious. **Infectious prostatitis** is caused by a virus, bacteria, or other organism. The choice of therapy depends on what type of organism is causing the problem. **Non-infectious prostatitis** means the prostate gland is inflamed, but there's no organism responsible for it. Non-infectious prostatitis is a diagnosis of exclusion. This means that all possible infectious causes have been ruled out. The cause of non-infectious prostatitis is not known, but could be due to a type of autoimmune condition. A variety of immune cells can enter the prostate gland and irritate it. The therapy for this type of prostatitis is difficult and doctors don't have any good drug options at this time.

The symptoms of non-infectious prostatitis include irritation on voiding, and discomfort in the anal or bladder region. These symptoms continue for a long time and can interfere with quality of life.

Studies with SP and Pygeum in the therapy of non-infectious prostatitis are limited, but have shown potential in reducing inflammatory responses (Marconi, 1986; Paubert-Braquet, 1994).

Another herb to consider is rye pollen extract. In 1991, Japanese researchers discovered that Cernilton (a rye pollen extract used in Europe) was an effective medicine in the therapy of prostatitis (Suzuki). No side effects were noted by the patients. Two years later, a group from Germany gave Cernilton, in a dose of 1 tablet three times a day for 6 months for the treatment of chronic prostatitis to 90 patients (Rugendorff, 1993). At the conclusion of the study, 78 percent showed improvement, while 36 percent were cured of their symptoms.

If your doctor determines that you have non-infectious prostatitis, and does not offer any adequate therapeutic options, it would certainly be worthwhile to give herbs a trial.

Does Cigarette Smoking Influence the Prostate?

Although it is believed that cigarette smoking is associated with a higher rate of prostate cancer, the limited research thus far does not indicate that smoking enlarges the prostate gland. In one study done in Turkey, middle-aged and older smokers were found to have a slightly smaller prostate gland than non-smokers (Kupeli, 1997). Perhaps smoking somehow influences levels of hormones within prostate tissue.

CHAPTER 15

Summary and Practical Recommendations

Saw palmetto and other herbal extracts have shown potential to be beneficial in easing symptoms of benign prostatic hyperplasia (BPH). Additional research may show them to play a role in hair, skin, and other tissues.

There are now a number of possible ways to treat BPH, including surgery (TURP-transurethral resection of the prostate) and pharmaceutical medicines, such as 5-alpha-reductase inhibitors and alphablockers. The extensive research with herbal products indicates that they are certainly worthwhile to try as first line therapy in easing symptoms of BPH. Generally, the drugs will work quicker but they have more potential to cause side effects. SP, Pygeum, and other natural compounds may work slower, but they are better tolerated, and often have fewer side effects. Please note that not everyone will respond to herbal medicines. Then again, not everyone responds to pharmaceutical drugs, either.

Before getting started on any medicines, have a thorough medical evaluation to make sure the genitourinary problems are due to BPH and not due to infection, bladder stones, or cancer. If the symptoms are due to an infection, antibiotics would most likely be curative.

If urinary symptoms are due to an enlarged prostate, there are four major approaches available. I'll discuss each one and the reader can decide which of these is the best option for his particular needs.

The Pharmaceutical Approach

This is mostly for individuals who have a severe case of prostate enlargement. Treatment would start with an alpha-blocker, such as Hytrin, in the evening. Keep in mind that alpha-blockers can cause low blood pressure and dizziness. The doctor may also prescribe a 5-alpha-reductase inhibitor such as Proscar.

This approach is the most common one taken by traditional American doctors.

The Pharmaceutical and Herbal Approach

This is again for individuals who have a severe case of prostate enlargement, or have a moderate case of enlargement but are impatient for quick relief. The pharmaceutical medicines generally start working quicker.

The recommendations stated above are followed as well as one of the approaches listed below. After a month or two, the patient could try gradually stopping the pharmaceutical medicines to see if the herbs are providing enough benefits.

The Herbal Step By Step Approach

If the doctor determines it is a mild or moderate case of BPH, it would be appropriate to give natural options a trial before proceeding to pharmaceutical agents.

- Under the guidance of a health care practitioner, start with saw palmetto extract at about 160 mg twice daily with meals. The bottle should say that the capsules contain 85 to 95% liposterolic extract.
- If insomnia, or shallow sleep are present, use melatonin 0.5 mg an hour or so before bed once, twice, or three times a week. Initially, melatonin can be taken nightly for two weeks before decreasing its frequency.
- Some improvement in symptoms can be expected within 2 to 6 weeks.
- If, after 6 weeks, the patient is not satisfied with the benefits, add extracts of Pygeum africanum to the regimen. The dose would be about 50 mg twice daily, with meals. Continue on this regimen for another month. Pygeum may work on the prostate in a different way, and the combination, therefore, could possible be cumulative.
- If, after a month, there is still no improvement, add extracts of stinging nettles. If extracts of nettles isn't available, buy the bulk form and make a tea from it by adding a teaspoon or two to a cup of boiled water. This can be drunk once or twice daily.
- If there is still no improvement, add beta-sitosterol at about 10 mg twice daily.
- Please keep in mind that the dosages I'm recommending are rough guidelines. Individuals may respond to lower dosages, or perhaps need higher amounts.
- Continue adding different herbs each month if the problems are not completely resolved. For

instance, the next herb to add would be rye pollen extracts. With time, add other herbs and nutrients such as pumpkin seeds, zinc, Epilobrium, and so on.

- By now there should be significant improvement. If there are still symptoms of BPH, it may be worthwhile to temporarily add a pharmaceutical agent, such as Hytrin, to the medical regimen. Of course, a doctor needs to be seen to get a prescription for this medicine. The usual starting dose is 1 mg in the evening.
- If, after a month, more help is needed, a trial with Proscar may be justified at 5 mg a day.
- If the symptoms have improved, gradually lower the dosage of the medicines and find the minimum dosage that provides benefits.
- As a last resort, if all herbal and pharmaceutical medicines have failed to provide adequate relief, surgery may be necessary. Hopefully, very few patients would need to resort to this option. My hope is that the growing use of natural supplements will dramatically lower the number of patients requiring surgical intervention.

The Shotgun Approach

If the sufferer doesn't really care to know which one of the herbs is working, and just wants quick relief, he may consider taking a few of the herbs mentioned above at the same time instead of adding each one separately. The advantage to this approach is that he may get faster relief. The disadvantage is that he won't know which one is helping him the most, or whether one of these herbs would have done the job by itself.

For the extremely impatient, who want much quicker relief from symptoms, a pharmaceutical medicine such as an alpha-blocker or a 5-alpha-reductase inhibitor such as Proscar can be started concurrently.

Dietary Suggestions

Of course, do not neglect the diet. Although the influence of food on prostate size growth is not quickly apparent, over time, what is eaten could make a significant difference.

* Include a wide variety of fresh fruits, vegetables, grains, and legumes in the diet. These may also reduce the risk for prostate cancer.
* Soy products have phytoestrogens which could be helpful
* Substitute green tea for sodas and coffee
* Decrease your consumption of red meat and fatty foods, and instead consume more fish.

Additionally

* Avoid the use of decongestants such as the ones found in cold medicines. Ephedrine and pseudoephedrine are some examples. Diet prescription pills can also be a problem.
* Avoid excessive alcohol
* Don't drink fluids at least two hours before bed. Drink a glass of water upon waking up in the morning in order to rehydrate the body.

References

Abbou CC, Hozneck A, McCarthy C. *Alfuzosin, a uroselective alpha blocker, versus Pygeum africanum, a plant extract: a randomized, controlled trial in patients with symptomatic benign prostatic hypertrophy (BPH).* Eur Urol 30 Suppl 2:77, 1996.

Adlercreutz H, Mazur W. *Phyto-oestrogens and western diseases.* Annals of Medicine 29:95–120, 1997. Excellent review article.

Adriazola Semino M, Lozano Ortega JL, et al. *Symptomatic treatment of benign hypertrophy of the prostate. Comparative study of prazosin and Serenoa repens* [in Spanish] Arch Esp Urol 45:211–213, 1995.

Andersen JT, Ekman P, Wolf H, et al. *Can finasteride reverse the progress of benign prostatic hyperplasia? A two-year placebo-controlled study.* Urology 46:631–637, 1995.

Andersson S, Russel DW. *Structural and biochemical properties of cloned and expressed human and rat steroid 5-alpha-reductases.* Proc Natl Acad Sci USA 87:3640–3644, 1990.

Authie D, Cauquil J. *A multicenter study of the efficacy of Permixon in daily practice.* C R Ther Pharmacol Clin 5(56):3–13, 1987.

Awad AB, Chen YC, Fink CS, Hemmessey T. *Beta-sitosterol inhibits HT-29 human colon cancer cell growth and alters mem-*

brane lipids. Anticancer Res 16:2797–2804, 1996. The effect of beta-sitosterol was studied on the growth of HT-29 human colon cell line. After supplementation with 16 microM beta-sitosterol for 9 days, cell growth was only one-third that of cells supplemented with equimolar concentration of cholesterol. The researchers say, "It is possible that the observed growth inhibition by beta-sitosterol may be mediated through the influence of signal transduction pathways that involve membrane phopholipids."

Bach D, Ebeling L. *Long-term drug treatment of benign prostatic hyperplasia-results of a prospective 3-year multicenter study using Sabal extract IDS 89.* Phytomedicine 3:105–111, 1996. Thanks to Donald Brown, N.D., for providing this article to me. "Pathohistological analysis of enucleated BPH tissue from 18 patients treated pre-operatively with IDS 89 and a placebo showed a significantly lower degree of glandular congestion and stromal edema in the prostate of the treated group (Helpap, 1995). In this respect, the increase in activity of the intra-prostatic enzyme, 3-alpha-hydroxysteroid-oxidoreductase following IDS 89 treatment is of particular interest. Enzyme-kinetic analysis of BPH tissue showed that the Vmax of 3-alpha-HSOR was significantly raised in the stroma of patients receiving the active preparation.

"Since the 3-alpha-SHOR possesses strong substrate affinity to the steroidal hormone DHT and to prostaglandins, the IDS 89-increased activity of this enzyme could be responsible for an increased metabolisation of DHT to 3-alpha-diol, as well as for an increased deactivation of prostaglandins in the prostate itself. The low deterioration rate seen in the three-year study could therefore be explained by a reduction of prostaglandin-mediated congestion or intraprostatic edema formation and thus prevention of subsequent sclerotic and fibrotic processes, as well as by a fall in androgen-mediated proliferation or elevated apoptosis."

Barlet A, Albrecht J, Aubert A, et al. *Efficacy of Pygeum africanum extract in the medical therapy of urination disorders due to benign prostatic hyperplasia: evaluation of objective and subjective parameters. A placebo-controlled double-blind multicenter study.* Wien Klin Wocheschr 102:667–673, 1990.

Berges RR. Windeler J, Trampisch HJ, Senge T. *Randomized, placebo-controlled, double-blind clinical trial of beta-sitosterol in patients with benign prostatic hyperplasia. Beta-sitosterol Study Group.* Lancet 345:1529–1532, 1995.

Berry SJ, Coffey DS, Walsh PC, Ewing LL. *The development of human benign prostatic hyperplasia with age.* J Urol 132:474–479, 1984.

Bjelfman C, Soderstrom TG, Brekkan E, Norlen BJ, Egevad L, Unge T, Andersson S, Rane A. *Differential gene expression of steroid 5-alpha-reductase 2 in core needle biopsies from malignant and benign prostatic tissue.* J Clin Endocrinol Metab 82:2210–2214, 1997. "The 5-alpha-2 specific messenger RNA (mRNA) levels were measured in 50 human prostate transrectal ultrasound-guided core biopsies obtained from 31 outpatients (median age 72, range 57–88 years) undergoing biopsy for diagnostic purposes. Significant differences were observed in the gene expression of 5-alpha-reductase 2 between cancerous and noncancerous tissue. In the 14 biopsies judged cancerous, the median 5-alpha-reductase 2 mRNA levels were 3.5 amol/ng total RNA compared with 12.0 amol/ng total RNA In the biopsies showing no cancer. The median 5-alpha-reductase 2 mRNA level in noncancerous tissue was thus 3.4 times higher than in the cancerous specimens."

Boyle P, Gould A, Rochrborn CG. *Prostate volume predicts outcome of treatment of benign prostatic hyperplasia with finasteride: meta-analysis of randomized clinical trials.* Urology 48:398–405, 1996.

Bracher F. *Phytotherapy of benign prostatic hyperplasia.* Urologe A, 36:10–7,1997. "Based on new study results, the use of phytopharmaceutical agents for the treatment of mild to moderate symptomatic BPH seems to be well justified."

Briley M, Carilla E, Roger A: *Inhibitory effect of Permixon on testosterone 5-alpha reductase activity of the rat ventral prostate.* Br J Pharmacol 83:401–410, 1984.

Bruchovsky N. *Comparison of the metabolites found in rat prostate following the in vivo administration of 7 natural androgens.* Endocrinology 89:1212–1218, 1971.

Bruchovsky N, Lesser B, van Doorn E, Craven S. *Hormonal effect on cell proliferation in rat prostate.* Vitam Horm 33:61—102, 1975.

Buck AC, Cox R, Rees RW Ebeling L, John A. *Treatment of outflow tract obstruction due to benign prostatic hyperplasia with the pollen extract Cernilton: A double-blind, placebo-controlled study.* Br J Urol 66:398–404, 1990.

Carani C, Salvioli V, Scuteri A, Borelli A, Baldini A, Granata AR, Marrama P. *Urological and sexual evaluation of treatment of benign prostatic disease using Pygeum africanum at high doses.* Arch Ital Urol Nefrol Androl 63:341–345, 1991. Pygeum africanum extract administration improved all the urinary parameters investigated. Prostatic echography revealed a reduction of peri-urethral edema. There were no significant differences between serum hormone levels of leutenizing hormone, follicular stimulating hormone and prolactin levels before and after therapy. There were also no differences in nocturnal penile tumescence and rigidity before and after therapy with Pygeum.

Carbin BE, Larsson B, Linahl O. *Treatment of benign prostatic hyperplasia with phytosterols.* Br J Urol, 66(6):639–641, 1990.

Carilla E, Briley M, Fauran F, et al. *Binding of Permixon, a new treatment for prostate benign hyperplasia, to the cytosolic* *androgen receptor in the rat prostate.* J Steroid Biochem 20:521–523, 1984.

Carraro JC, Raynaud JP, Koch G, Chisholm GD, Di Silverio F, Teillac P, Da Silva FC, Cauquil J, Chopin DK, Hamdy FC, Hanus M, Hauri D, Kalinteris A, Marencak J, Perier A, Perrin P. *Comparison of phytotherapy (Permixon) with finasteride in the treatment of benign prostate hyperplasia: a randomized international study of 1,098 patients.* The Prostate 29:231–240, 1996. Pierre Fabre Medicaments, the makers of Permixon, were involved in organizing this study.

Casarosa C, Cosci di Coscio M, Fratta M. *Lack of effects of a liposterolic extract of Serenoa repens on plasma levels of testosterone, follicle-stimulating hormone, and luteinizing hormone.* Clin Ther 10:585, 1988.

Champault G, Patel J, Bonnard A. *A double-blind trial of an extract of the plant Serenoa repens in benign prostatic hyperplasia.* Br J Clin Pharmac 18:461–462, 1984.

Champault G, Bonnard A, Cauquil J, Patel JC. *Medical treatment of the prostatic adenoma: A controlled test of PA 109 (Permixon: Serenoa repens extract) vs. placebo in 100 patients.* Ann Urol 6: 407–410, 1984.

Chang JL, Char GY. Benign hypertrophy of prostate. Chin Med J [Engl] 50:1707–1722, 1936.

Cunha GR. *Epithelial-stromal interaction in development of the urogenital tract.* Int Rev Cytol 47:137–194, 1994. DHT made in the prostate gland by the 5-alpha-reductase type 2 enzyme contributes to the induction, proliferation, and differentiation of the adjacent prostatic epithelial cells.

Dai R, Jacobson, KA, Robinson RC, Friedman FK. *Differential effects of flavonoids on testosterone-metabolizing cytochrome P450s.* Life Sciences 61:7:75–80, 1997.

Dalton DP, Lee C, Huprikar S, et al. *Non-androgenic role of testis in enhancing ventral prostate growth in rates.* Prostate 16:225–233, 1990.

Dathe G, Schmid H. *Phytotherapy of benign prostate hyperplasia with Serenoa repens extract (Permixon).* Urologe Ausg B 31(5):220–223, 1991.

Denis LJ. *Editorial review of "Comparison of phytotherapy (Permixon) with finasteride in the treatment of benign prostate hyperplasia: A randomized international study of 1098 patients.* The Prostate 29:241–242, 1996.

Descotes JL, Rumbaed JJ, Deschaseaux P, et al. *Placebo-controlled evaluation of the efficacy and tolerability of Permixon in benign prostatic hyperplasia after exclusion of placebo responders.* Clin Drug Invest 9:291–297, 1995.

Desgrandchamps F. *Clinical relevance of growth factor antagonists in the treatment of benign prostatic hyperplasia.* Eur Urol 32:1:28–31, 1997.

Di Silverio F, D'Eramo G, Lubrano C, Flammia P, et al. *Evidence that Serenoa repens extract displays an antiestrogenic activity in prostatic tissue of benign prostatic hypertrophy.* Eur Urol 21:309–314, 1992. Serenoa repens extract was able to inhibit both nuclear estrogen receptors and nuclear androgen receptors in prostate tissue samples of BPH patients. "Whatever could be the mechanism of action of S. repens extract, its antiestrogenic effect is well documented, so that we may assume that this drug interferes at noncytotoxic doses with the molecular mechanisms involved in cell growth."

Di Silverio F, Sciarra A, D'Eramo G, Casale P, Di Nicola S, Buscarini M, Sciarra F. *Response of tissue androgen and epidermal growth factor concentrations to the long-term administration of Serenoa Repens (Permixon), finasteride and flutamide to BPH patients.* Eur Urol 30, Suppl 2:96, 1996. "Flutamide, finasteride and Serenoa repens decrease the local androgen support and the production of growth factor mainly in the periurethral zone. These findings further support the assumption that DHT and EGF (epidermal growth factor) are involved in the development of clinical BPH."

Dreikorn K, Schonhofer PS. *Status of phytotherapeutic drugs in treatment of prostatic hyperplasia.* Urologe A, 34(2):119–129, 1995. There has been an increase in the use herbal products in Germany in the therapy of BPH. Sales in 1995 were 220 million Marks. The preparations most commonly used are extracts of hypoxis rooperi, the roots of the stinging nettle, the fruits of saw palmetto, pumpkin seeds and rye pollen.

Droller MJ. *Medical approaches in the management of prostatic disease.* British J Urol 79S:42–52, 1997.

Ducrey B, Marston A, Gohring S, Hartmann RW, Hostettmann K. *Inhibition of 5-alpha-reductase by the ellagitannins Oenothein A and Oenothein B from Epilobium species.* Planta Medica 63:111–114, 1997.

Dutkiewicz S. *Zinc and magnesium serum levels in patients with benign prostatic hyperplasia (BPH) before and after prazosin therapy.* Mater Med Pol 27:15–17, 1995.

Dutkiewicz S. *Usefulness of Cernilton in the treatment of benign prostatic hyperplasia.* Int Urol Nephrol 28:49–53, 1996.

Ebbinghaus KD. *Efficacy of Permixon in the treatment of benign prostatic hyperplasia* [in German]. Journal Für Urologie und Urogynakologie 2:17–21, 1995.

Ekman P. *BPH epidemiology and risk factors.* Prostate, S2:23–31, 1989.

Eri L, Tveter K. *Alpha-blockade in the treatment of symptomatic benign prostatic hyperplasia.* J Urol 154:923–934, 1995.

Eri L, Tveter K. *Treatment of benign prostatic hyperplasia: A pharmacological perspective.* Drugs and Aging 10(2):107–118, 1997.

Fabricius PG, Weizert P, et al. *Efficacy of once-a-day terazosin in benign prostatic hyperplasia: a randomized, double-blind placebo-controlled clinical trial.* Prostate Suppl 3:85–93, 1990.

Fahim AT, Abd-el Fattah AA, Agha AM, Gad MZ. *Effect of pumpkin-seed oil on the level of free radical scavengers induced during adjuvant-arthritis in rats.* Pharmacol Res 31(1):73–79, 1995.

Fahim MS, Wang M, Sutcu MF, Fahim Z. *Zinc arginine, a 5-alpha-reductase inhibitor, reduces rat ventral prostate weight and DNA without affecting testicular function.* Andrologia 25:369–375, 1993. This paper mentions a study where 1 ml of 100 mg zinc arginine was injected into each lateral lobe of the human prostate gland of patients with BPH. All of the patients experienced a sensation of swelling at the area of injection for 1–4 days; no other reactions were observed. The results showed significant decrease in symptoms of obstruction, an increase in urinary flow, and a decrease in prostatic volume.

Fitzpatrick J, Lynch T. *Phytotherapeutic agents in the management of symptomatic benign prostatic hyperplasia.* Advances in Benign Prostatic Hyperplasia 22:2; 407–412, 1995.

Garraway W, Russell E, Lee RJ, et al. *Impact of previously unrecognized benign prostatic hyperplasia on the daily activities of middle-aged and elderly men.* Br J Gen Pract 43:318–321, 1993.

Gilad E, Matzkin H, Zisapel N. *Interplay between sex steroids and melatonin in regulation of human benign prostate epithelial cell growth.* J Clin Endo and Metab 82:2535–2541, 1997.

Giovannucci E, Ascherio A, Rimm E, et al. *Intake of carotenoids and retinol in relation to risk of prostate cancer.* J Natl Cancer Inst 87:1767–1776, 1995.

Gormley GJ, Stoner E, Bruskewitz RC, et al. *The effect of finasteride in men with benign prostatic hyperplasia.* N Engl J Med 327:1185–1191, 1992.

Grasso M, Montesano A, Buonaguidi A, Castelli M, Lania C, Rigatti P, Rocco F, Cesana BM, Borghi C. *Comparative effects* of alfuzosin versus Serenoa repens in the treatment of symptomatic benign prostatic hyperplasia. Arch Esp Urol 48:97–103, 1995.

Grayhack JT. *Pituitary factors influencing growth of the prostate.* Natl Cancer Inst Monogr 12:198–199, 1963.

Gu FI, Xia TL, Kong XT. *Preliminary study of the frequency of benign prostatic hyperplasia and prostatic cancer in China.* Urology 44:699–691, 1994.

Guess HA, Jacobsen SJ, Girman CJ, et al. *The role of community-based longitudinal studies in evaluating treatment effects. Example: benign prostatic hyperplasia.* Med Care 33:AS26–35, 1995.

Gutilerrez M, Hidalgo A, Cantabrana B. *Spasmolytic activity of a lipidic extract from Sabal serrulata fruits: further study of the mechanisms underlying this activity.* Planta Med 62:507–511, 1996. Results suggest that the spasmolytic effect of lipidic extract from S. serrulata fruits could be partially due to sodium/calcium exchanger activation and interference with intracellular calcium mobilization, and point to cAMP as a possible mediator.

Habib FK, Ross M, Buck AC, et al. *In vitro evaluation of the pollen extract Cernilton T-60 in the regulation of prostate cell growth.* Br J Urol 66:393–397, 1990.

Habib FK, Ross M. Lewenstein A, Zhang X, Jaton JC. *Identification of a prostate inhibitory substance in a pollen extract.* Prostate 26(3):133–139, 1995.

Helpap B, Oehler U, Weisser H, Bach D, Ebeling L. *Morphology of benign prostatic hyperplasia after treatment with Sabal extract IDS 89 or placebo.* J Urol Pathol 3:175–182, 1995.

Hiermann A, Reidlinger M, Juan H, Semetz W. *Isolation of the antiphlogistic principle from Epilobium augustifolium.* Planta Med 57(4):357–360, 1991.

Hiermann A, Bucar F. *Studies of Epilobium augustifolium extracts on growth of accessory sexual organs in rats.* J. Ethnopharmacol 55(3):179–183, 1997.

Horst H, Buck A, Adam K. *Orally administered melatonin stimulates the 3 alpha/beta hydroxy steroid oxidoreductase but not the 5-alpha-reductase in the ventral prostate and seminal vesicles of pinealectomized rats.* Experientia 38:968–970, 1982.

Hyrb DJ, Khan MS, Romas NA, Rosner W. *The effect of extracts of the roots of the stinging nettle (Urtica dioica) on the interaction of SHBG with its receptor on human prostatic membranes.* Planta Med 61:31–32, 1995. "Four substances contained in Uritica dioica were examined: an aqueous extract; an alcoholic extract; U dioica agglutinin, and stigmasta-4-en-3-one. Of these, only the aqueous extract was active. It inhibited the binding of 125I-SHBG to its receptor. The inhibition was dose related, starting at about 0.6 mg/ml and completely inhibited at 10 mg/ml."

Huggins C, Stevens R, Hodges CV. *Studies on prostate cancer. The effect of castration on advanced carcinoma of the prostate gland.* Arch Surg 43:209–233, 1997.

Humiczewska M, Hermach U, Put A. *The effect of the pollen extracts quercitin and cernitin on the liver, lungs, and stomach of rats intoxicated with ammonium fluoride.* Folia Biol (Krakow) 42:3–4:157–166, 1994.

Jenkins EP, Andersson S, Imperato-McGinley, et al. *Genetic and pharmacologic evidence for more than one human steroid 5-alpha-reductase.* J Clin Invest 89:293–300, 1992.

Juniewicz PE, Berry SJ, Coffey DS, Strandberg JD, Ewing LL: *Requirement of testis in establishing sensitivity of canine prostate to develop benign prostatic hyperplasia.* J Urol 152:996–1001, 1994.

Kolonel LN. *Nutrition and prostate cancer.* Cancer Causes Control 7:83, 1996. "Whereas a clear association with obesity has not been shown, a positive relationship to muscle mass, though not yet established conclusively, further suggests the importance of androgens in this cancer."

Kondas J, Philipp V, Dioszeghy G. *Sabal serrulata extract in the management of symptoms of prostatic hypertrophy.* Orv Hetil 138:419–421, 1997.

Krieg M, Bartsch W, Thomsen M, Voigt KD. *Androgens and estrogens: Their interaction with stroma and epithelium of human benign prostatic hyperplasia and normal prostate.* J Steroid Biochem 19:155–161, 1983.

Krzeski T, Kazon M, Borkowski A, Witeska A, Kuczera J. *Combined extracts of Urtica dioica and Pygeum africanum in the treatment of benign prostatic hyperplasia: double-blind comparison of two doses.* Clin Ther 15:1011–1020, 1993.

Kupeli B, Soygur T, Aydos K, Ozdiler E, Kupeli S. *The role of cigarette smoking in prostatic enlargement.* British J Urol 80:201–204, 1997.

Kvanta E. *Sterols in pollen.* Acta Chem Scand 22:2161–2165, 1968.

Laure JP, Morfin RF, Charles JF. *Zinc in the human prostate.* J Urol (Paris) 91(7):463–468, 1985.

Laudon M, Gilad E, Matzkin H, Braf Z, Zisapel N. *Putative melatonin receptors in benign human prostate tissue.* J Clin Endocrinol Metab 81:1336–1342, 1996.

Leake A, Chisholm GD, Habib FK. *The effect of zinc on the 5-alpha-reduction of testosterone by the hyperplastic human prostate gland.* J Steroid Biochem 20(2):651–655, 1984.

Lee C, Kozlowski J, Grayhack J. *Intrinsic and extrinsic factors controlling benign prostatic growth.* The Prostate 31:131–138, 1997.

Lee C, Prins GS, Henneberry MO, Grayhack JT. *Effect of estradiol on the rat prostate in the presence and absence of testosterone and pituitary.* J Androl 2:293–299, 1981.

Lehle C, Delos S, Guirou O, et al. *Human prostate steroid 5-alpha-reductase isoforms—a comprehensive study of selective inhibitors.* J Steroid Biochem Mol Biol 54:273–279, 1995.

Lepor H, Wiliford WO, Barry MJ, et al. *The efficacy of terazosin, finasteride, or both, in benign prostatic hyperplasia.* N Engl J Med 335:553–559, 1996.

Lesuisse D, Berjonneau J, Ciot C, et al. *Determination of Oenothein B as the active 5-alpha-reductase-inhibiting principle of the folk medicine Epilobium parviflorum.* J Natural Products 59:490–492, 1996.

Liao S, Umekita Y, Guo J, et al. *Growth inhibition and regression of human prostate and breast tumors in athymic mice by tea epigallocatechin gallate.* Cancer Lett 96:239–243, 1995.

Liao S, Hiipakka RA. Biochem Biophys Res Commun 214, 833–838, 1995.

Linassier C, Pierre M, Le Pecq JB, Pierre J. *Mechanisms of action in NIH-3T3 cells of genistein, an inhibitor of EGF receptor tyrosine kinase activity.* Biochem Pharmacol 39:187, 1989.

Liu Y, Franklin RB, Costello LC. *Prolactin and testosterone regulation of mitochondrial zinc in prostate epithelial cells.* The Prostate 30:26–32, 1997. "Our results support the concept that mitochondrial zinc is an inhibitor of m-aconitase and citrate oxidation, and that prolactin and testosterone regulation of mitochondrial zinc provides a mechanism for their regulation of citrate oxidation in citrate-producing prostate epithelial cells."

Magdy El-Sheikh M, Dakka MR, Saddique A. *The effect of Permixon on androgen receptors.* Acta Obstet Gynecol Scand 67:397–399, 1988.

Mandressi S, Tarallo U, Maggioni A, et al. *Medical treatment of benign prostatic hyperplasia: efficacy of the extract of Serenoa repens (Permixon) compared to that of the extract of Pygeum africanum and a placebo.* Urologia 50:752–758, 1983.

Marconi M, D'Angelo L, Del Vecchio, A. Caravaggi M, et al. *Anti-inflammatory action of Pygeum africanum extract in the rat.* Farmaci & Terapia 3:135, 1986.

McConnell JD, Wilson J, George FW, Geller J, Pappas F, Stoner E. *Finasteride, an inhibitor of 5-alpha-reductase, suppresses prostatic dihydrotestosterone in men with benign prostatic hyperplasia.* J Clin Endocrinol Metab 74:505, 1992.

Mebust WK, Holtgrewe HL, Cockett AT, et al. *Transurethral prostatectomy: immediate and postoperative complications: a cooperative study of 13 participating institutions evaluating 3885 patients.* J Urol 141:243–247, 1989.

Miyamoto KI, Nomura M, Sasakura M, et al. Biol Pharm Bull 16:379–387, 1993.

Modern Medicine, volume 65, page 40, May 1997.

Monda JM, Oesterling JE. *Subspecialty clinics: urology. Medical treatment of benign prostatic hyperplasia. 5-alpha-reductase inhibitors and alpha-adrenergic antagonists.* Mayo Clin Proc 68:670–679, 1993.

Murkovic M, Hillebrand A, Winkler J, Leitner E, Pfannhauser W. *Variability of fatty acid content in pumpkin seeds.* Z Lebensm Unters Forsch 204:216–219, 1996.

Nicoletti M, Galeffi C, Messana I, Marini-Bettolo GB. *Hypoxidaceae. Medicinal uses and the norlignan constituents.* J Ethnopharmacology 36:95–101, 1992.

Nishi N, Matuo Y, Kunitomi K, Takenaka I, Usami M, Kotake T, Wada F. *Comparative analysis of growth factors in normal and pathologic human prostates.* Prostate 13:38, 1988.

Novelli EL, Rodriguez NL, Santos CX, Martinez FE, Novelli JL. *Toxic effects of alcohol intake on prostate of rats.* Prostate 31:37–41, 1997.

Obertreis B, Giller K, Teucher T, Behnke B, Schmitz H. *Antiphlogistic effects of Urtica dioica folia extract in comparison to caffeic malic acid.* Drug Res 46:52–56, 1996.

Osterling JE, Roy J, Agha A, Shown T, Krarup T, Johansen T, et al. *Biologic variability of prostate-specific antigen and its usefulness as a marker for prostate cancer: effects of finasteride.* Urology 50:13–18, 1997.

Oliviera S, Lee IM. *Is exercise beneficial in the prevention of prostate cancer?* Sport Med 23(5):271–278, 1997.

Paubert-Braquet M, Cave A, Hocquemiller R, Delacroix D, Dupont C, Hedef N, Borgeat P. *Effect of Pygeum africanum extract on A23187-stimulated production of lipoxygenase metabolites from human polymorphonuclear cells.* J Lipid Mediat Cell Signal 9(3):285–290, 1994. Infiltration by inflammatory cells may be involved in the development of BPH. Certain of these cell types, such as macrophages, are known to produce chemotactic mediators including leukotrienes, and thus may contribute to the development of the disease. In order to investigate the potential effect of Pygeum extract on arachidonate metabolism, the researchers examined its effect in vitro on leukotriene (LT) synthesis in human polymorphonuclear cells stimulated with the calcium ionophore A23187. Pygeum inhibited the production of 5-lipoxygenase metabolites. The researchers state, "The ability of Pygeum to antagonize 5-lipxygenase metabolite production may contribute, at least in part, to its therapeutic activity in inflammatory component of BPH."

Paubert-Braquet M, Janssen DH, Servent N, et al. *Permixon (lipido sterolic extract of Serenoa repens (LSESr) inhibits b-FGF and EGF-induced proliferation of human prostate organotypic cell lines* (abstract). Pharmacol Res 31:Suppl:69, 1995.

Paubert-Braquet M, Richardson F, Servent-Saez N, Gordon WC, Monge MC, Bazan NG, Authie D, Braquet P. *Effect of Serenoa repens extract (Permixon) on estradiol/testosterone-induced experimental prostate enlargement in the rat.* Pharmacol Res 34:3/4, 1996. "*Serenoa repens* extract administration does not equally reduce the weight of the different parts of the rat experimentally enlarged prostate, as the maximal effect was noted for the dorsal lobe, the lateral lobes are less sensitive to the extract, whereas the effect on the ventral lobe is very weak."

Pinelli A, Trivulzio S. *Antiprostatic effect associated with zinc depletion in cimetidine-treated rats.* Pharmacol Res Commun 20(4):329–335, 1988.

Plosker G, Brogden R. *Sereno repens (Permixon): A review of its pharmacology and therapeutic efficacy in benign prostatic hyperplasia.* Drugs and Aging 9(5):379–395, 1996. An excellent review of *in Vitro* studies, *in Vivo* studies in animal models and humans, pharmacokinetic properties, mechanisms of action, and therapeutic efficacy.

Ragab A, Ragab-Thomas JMF, Delhon A, et al. *Effects of Permixon on phopholipase A2 activity and on arachidonic acid metabolism in cultured prostatic cells.* New trends in BPH Etiopathogenesis 293–296, 1987.

Ravenna R, Di Silverio F, Russo MA, Salvatori L, Morgante E, Morrone S, Cardillo MR, Russo A, Frati L, Gulino A, Petrangeli E. *Effects of the lipidosterolic extract of Serenoa repens (Permixon) on human prostatic cell lines.* The Prostate 29:219–230, 1996. The effects of Permixon on two prostatic cell lines differing on androgen responsiveness were tested. 1) PC3 (bone metastasis of prostatic carcinoma), which expresses a very low level of wild-type androgen receptor and is unresponsive to androgens, glucocorticoids, and fibroblast growth factors. 2) LNCaP (lymph node carcinoma of the prostate), which maintains several characteristics of primary human prostatic carcinoma, such as the dependence on androgens and the production of acid phosphatase.

Permixon showed a higher toxicity on the more differentiated, hormone-dependent LNCaP cell line with respect to PC3 cells. This may indicate that in some way hormone dependency makes cells more susceptible to the action of the drug. Electron microscope studies seem to indicate that cellular permeability to the liposterolic plant extract is higher in LNCaP cells.

Rhodes L, Primka R, Berman C, Vergult G, Gabriel M, Pierre-Malice M, Gibelin B. *Comparison of finasteride (Proscar), a 5-alpha reductase-inhibitor, and various commercial plant extracts in In vitro and In vivo 5-alpha reductase inhibition.* The Prostate 22:43–51, 1993.

Robinette CL. *Sex-hormone-induced inflammation and fibromuscular proliferation in the rat lateral prostate.* Prostate 12:271–286, 1988.

Romics I, Schmitz H, Frang D. *Experience in treating benign prostatic hypertrophy with Sabal serrulata for one year.* International Urology and Nephrology 25:565–569, 1993. Forty-two patients with BPH were treated with the Sabal extract Strogen forte for 12 months. The obstructive symptoms, residual volume, mean and maximum flow rates improved significantly by the 6th therapeutic month at the latest. Side effects were not observed.

Rosner W. *Plasma steroid-binding proteins.* Endocrinol Metab Clin North Am 20:697–720, 1991.

Rugendorff EW, Weidner W, Ebeling L, Buck AC. *Results of treatment with pollen extract (Cernilton N) in chronic prostatitis and prostatodynia.* Br J Urol, 71:433–438, 1993. Those with complicating factors, such as urethral strictures, prostatic calculi, and bladder neck sclerosis, did not improve.

Russell, Alice. *Poisonous plants of North Carolina.* 1997. North Carolina State University.

Ruud Bosch JLH. *Conservative non-instrumental treatment of benign prostatic hyperplasia.* Urol res 25[Suppl 2]:S107–S114, 1997.

Sanda MG, Doehring CB, Binkowitz B, Beaty TH, Partin AW, Hale E, Stoner E, Walsh PC. *Clinical and biological characteristics of familial benign prostatic hyperplasia.* J Urol 157:876–879, 1997.

Schneider HJ, Honold E, Masuhr T. *Treatment of benign prostatic hyperplasia: Results of a treatment study with the phytogenic combination of Sabal extract WS 1473 and Urtica extract WS 1031 in urologic specialty practices.* Fortschr Med 113:37–40, 1995.

Sherwood ER, Fong C, Lee C, Koslowsky JM. *Basic fibroblast growth factor: a potential mediator of stromal growth in the human prostate.* Endocrinology 130:2955, 1992.

Shimada H, Tyler V, McLaughlin J. *Biologically active acylglycerides from the berries of saw palmetto (Serenoa repens).* J Nat Prod 60, 417–418, 1997. Extracts of Serenoa repens are prepared by supercritical fluid extraction with CO_2 or by extracting with hexane. "Monolaurin and monomyristin showed moderate biological activities in the brine shrimp lethality test and against renal (A-498) and pancreatic (PACA-2) human tumor cells; borderline cytotoxicity was exhibited against human prostatic (PC-3) cells."

Shirima K, Furuya T, Takeo Y, Shimizu K, Maekawa K. *Direct effect of melatonin on the accessory sexual organs in pinealectomized male rats kept in constant darkness.* J Endocrinol 95:87–94, 1982.

Silver RF, Wiley EK, Thigpen AE, Guileyardo JM, McConnell JD, Russell DW. *Cell type specific expression of steroid 5-alpha-reductase 2.* J Urol 152:438–442, 1994. The 5-alpha-reductase 2 enzyme is located mainly in the stromal fraction of the prostate.

Sitteree PK, Wilson JD. *Dihydrotestosterone of prostatic hypertrophy. The formation and content of dihydrotestosterone in the hypertrophic state of man.* J Clin Invest 49:1737–1745, 1970.

Smith RH, Memon A, Smart CJ, Dewbury K. *The value of Permixon in benign prostatic hypertrophy.* British J Urol 58:36–40, 1986.

Sriuilai W, Withyacitumroarnku, B. *Stereological changes in rat ventral prostate induced by melatonin.* J Pineal Res 6:111–119, 1989.

Stoner E, and Members of the Finasteride Study Group: *Three-year safety and efficacy data on the use of finasteride in the treatment of benign prostatic hyperplasia.* Urology 43:284–294, 1994.

Strauch S, Perles P, Vergult et al. *Comparison of finasteride (Proscar) and Serenoa repens (Permixon) in the inhibition of 5-alpha reductase in healthy male volunteers.* Eur Urol 26:247–252, 1994.

Sultan C, Terraza A, Devillier C, Carilla E, Briley M, Loire C, Descomps B. *Inhibition of androgen metabolism and binding by a liposterolic extract of serenoa repens B in human foreskin fibroblasts.* J Steroid Biochem 20:(1):515–519, 1984. "The present studies show that SP extract inhibits 5-alpha-reductase, 3-ketosteroid reductase and receptor binding of androgens in cultured human foreskin fibroblasts. As the search for the ideal antiandrogen continues, SP extract appears to be a new type of antiandrogenic compound as therapeutics for the treatment of benign prostatic hypertrophy, hirsutism and so forth."

Suzuki T, Kurokawa K, Mashimo T, Takezawa Y, Kobayashi D, et al. *Clinical effect of Cernilton in chronic prostatis.* Hinyokika Kiyo 38:489–494, 1992.

Szutrely HP. *Changes in the echostructure of prostatic adenoma during drug therapy.* Med Klin [Prax], 77(18):42–46, 1982.

Tanner, George, Mullahey, J Jeffrey, Maehr, David. *Saw palmetto: an ecologically and economically important native palm.* University of Florida, Institute of Food and Agricultural Sciences, 1997. As posted on their web site. IFAS Circular WEC-109. http://arc.imok.ufl.edu/mullahey.html

Tenover J. *Prostates, pates, and pimples. The potential medical uses of steroid 5-alpha-reductase inhibitors.* Endocrinology and Metabolism Clinics in North America 20:4;893–903, 1991.

Theyer G, Kramer G, Assmann I, Sherwood E, et al. *Phenotypic characterization of infiltrating leukocytes in benign prostatic hyperplasia.* Lab Invest 66:96–107, 1992.

Toth I, Szecsi M, Julesz J, Faredin I, Behnke B. *In vitro inhibition of testicular delta 5-3 beta-hydroxysteroid dehydrogenase and prostatic 5-alpha-reductase activities in rats and humans by Strogen forte extract.* Int Urol Nephrol 28:337–348, 1996. Strogen forte proved to be a direct inhibitor of rat testicular delta 5-3 beta-HSD and human testicular delta 5-3 beta-HSD. In addition, Strogen forte was found to inhibit prostatic 5-alpha-reductase in rats and humans.

Tvedt KE, Halgunset J, Kopstad G, Haugen OA. *Intracellular distribution of calcium and zinc in normal, hyperplastic, and neoplastic prostate. X-ray microanalysis of freeze-dried cryosections.* Prostate 15(1):41–51, 1989.

Vacher P, Prevarskaya N, et al. *The lipidosterolic extract from Serenoa repens interferes with prolactin receptor signal transduction.* J Biomed Sci 2:357–365, 1995.

Vahlensieck W, Fabricius PG, Hell U. *Drug therapy of benign prostatic hyperplasia.* Fortschr Med, 114:407–411, 1996.

Wager H, Willer F, Kreher B. *Biologically active compounds from the aqueous extract of Urtica dioica.* Planta Med 55(5):452–454, 1989. A polysaccharide fraction was isolated from the water extracts of the roots of Urtica. This lectin was found to stimulate the proliferation of human lymphocytes.

Walsh PC, Hutchins GM, Ewing LL. *Tissue content of dihydrotestosterone in human prostatic hyperplasia is not supranormal.* J Clin Invest 72:1772–1777, 1983.

Weisser H, Behnke B, Helpap B, Bach D, Krieg M. *Enzyme activities in tissue of human benign prostatic hyperplasia after three months' treatment with the Sabal serrulata extract IDS 89 (Strogen) or placebo.* Eur Urol 31:97–101, 1997. This double-blind, placebo-controlled clinical trial with the S. Serrulata extract IDS 89 given to men with BPH for 3 months revealed significant biochemical changes at the cellular level of BPH tissue. Prostate tissue samples were taken during a suprapubic prostatectomy. However, the alterations were moderate, their biochemical causes and consequences regarding the pathophysiology of BPH remain uncertain.

West DW, Slattery ML, Robison LM, French TK, Mahoney AW. *Adult dietary intake and prostate cancer risk in Utah: a case-control study with special emphasis on aggressive tumors.* Cancer Causes Control 2:85–94, 1991.

Wilde M, Fitton A, Sorkin EM. *Terazosin: a review of its pharmacodynamic properties, and therapeutic potential in benign prostatic hyperplasia.* Drugs and Aging 3:258–277, 1993.

Wingo PA, Tong T, Bolden S, Parker SL. *Cancer statistics,* CA 47:5–27, 1995.

Wright ET, Chmiel JS, Grayhack Jt, Schaeffer AJ. *Prostatic fluid inflammation in prostatitis.* J Urol 152:2300–2303, 1994.

Wu JP, Gu FL. *The prostate 41–65 years post-castration: An analysis of 26 eunuchs.* Chin Med J 100:271–272, 1987.

Yablonsky F, Nicolas V, Riffaud JP, Bellamy F. *Antiproliferative effect of Pygeum africanum extract on rat prostatic fibroblasts.* J of Urology 157:2381–2387, 1997. "These results show that Pygeum africanum is a potent inhibitor of rat prostatic fibroblast proliferation in response to direct activators of protein kinase C, the defined growth factors bFGF, EGF, IGF-I, and the complex mixture of mitogens in serum depending on the concentration used. PKC activation appears to be an important growth factor-mediated signal transduction for this agent. These data suggest that therapeutic effect of Pygeum africanum may be due at least in part to the inhibition of growth factors responsible for the prostatic overgrowth in man."

Yasumoto R, Kawanishi H, Tsujino T, Tsujita M, Nishisaka N, Horri A, Kishimoto T. *Clinical evaluation of long-term treatment using cernitin pollen extract in patients with benign prostatic hyperplasia.* Clin Ther 17:82–87, 1995.

Yu EY, Siegal JA, Meyer GE, Ji XR, Ni XZ, Brawer MK. *Histologic differences in benign prostate hyperplasia between Chinese and American men.* The Prostate 31:175–179, 1997.

Zhang X, Habib FK, Ross M, Burger U, Lewenstein A, Rose K, Jaton JC. *Isolation and characterization of a cyclic hydroxamic acid from a pollen extract, which inhibits cancerous cell growth in vitro.* J Med Chem 38:735–738, 1995.

Zhang J, Hess MW, Thurnher M, Hobisch A, Radmayr C, Cronauer MV, Hittmair A, Culig Z, Bartsch G, Klocker H. *Human prostatic smooth muscle cells in culture: estradiol enhances expression of smooth muscle cell-specific markers.* The Prostate 30:117–129, 1997.

Zhang X, Ouyang JZ, Zhang YS, Tayalla B, Zhou XC, Zhou SW. *Effect iof the extracts of pumpkin seeds on the urodynamic of rabbits: an experimental study.* J Tongji Med Univ, 14(4):235–238, 1994.

About the Author

Ray Sahelian, M.D., is a physician certified by the American Board of Family Practice. He obtained a Bachelor of Science degree in nutrition from Drexel University and completed his doctoral training at Thomas Jefferson Medical School, both in Philadelphia.

A popular and respected physician and medical writer, Dr. Sahelian is internationally recognized as a moderate voice in the evaluation of herbs, nutrients and hormones. He has been seen on numerous television programs including *NBC Nightly News, CBS This Morning, NBC Weekend, CNN, Geraldo, Hard Copy, Extra, Dini Petty Show* (Canada), *MBC* (Korea), *Zone Interdite* (France); quoted by countless major magazines such as *Modern Maturity, Newsweek, Men's Health, Cosmopolitan, Men's Journal, Modern Medicine, Allure, Health, Ms. Fitness;* and quoted in hundreds of newspapers including *USA Today, USA Weekend, Los Angeles Times, The Washington Post, The Miami Herald, American Medical News,* and *Le Monde* (France). His articles have appeared in numerous health magazines. Millions of listeners from over 3,000 radio stations nationwide have heard him discuss the latest research on health and medical topics.

Dr. Sahelian is the Editor of *Longevity Research Update,* and a nationally-known lecturer. He is also the 700,000 plus bestselling author of *Melatonin: Nature's Sleeping Pill, DHEA: A Practical Guide, Creatine: Nature's Muscle Builder, Pregnenolone: Nature's Feel Good Hormone, Glucosamine: Nature's Arthritis Remedy, St. John's Wort, CoQ10, Kava, Stevia,* and *Lipoic Acid.* His books have been translated into French, Germany, Italian, Spanish, Korean, Chinese, Japanese, and Russian. See www.raysahelian.com for latest updates.

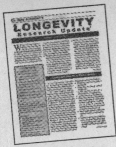

No hype, just the facts

Longevity Research Update
Eight-page newsletter

Research in hormone replacement therapy, nutrition, and longevity is accelerating. If you wish to keep up with the latest information on melatonin, DHEA, pregnenolone, estrogen, progesterone, testosterone, growth hormone, other hormones, creatine, glucosamine, saw palmetto, herbs, and other supplements, then this is the right newsletter for you. Dr. Sahelian and his staff constantly scan hundreds of new articles published in prestigious journals all over the world. They present a balanced interpretation of the important findings. No hype, just the facts.

The newsletter is published in January, April, July and October. Visit the web site: www.raysahelian.com for the latest updates!

For the latest updates, visit the web site: www.raysahelian.com

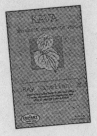

Kava: Nature's Answer to Anxiety

This booklet offers a well-rounded definition of kava, an herb used for anxiety and nervous tension. The author explains the history of kava, its many uses, the landmark study that confirms it efficacy, and important cautions.

Paperback, 32 pages • $3.95 (Includes shipping & handling)

St. John's Wort: Nature's Feel-Good Herb

Medical studies have shown St. John's wort to be a good alternative to prescription antidepressants, as discussed in *Newsweek* and on the popular television show *20/20*. This definitive guide discusses the practical uses of the herb, along with its safety and how it interacts with medicines and nutrients. Dr. Sahelian is an authority and has been seen on *NBC Nightly News*.

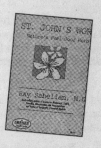

Paperback, 32 pages • $3.95 (Includes shipping & handling)

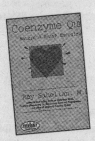

Coenzyme Q10: Nature's Heart Energizer

This definitive guide reviews the practical uses of this antioxidant nutrient, the proper dosages along with its safety and how it interacts with other supplements.

Paperback, 27 pages • $3.95 (Includes shipping & handling)

plus new books Lipoic Acid and Stevia.

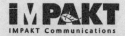

IMPAKT Communications

Available at your local health food store or by calling:
U.S. 1-800-477-2995 or 310-821-2409, Canada 1-888-292-2229 or 604-421-5887

Additional books of interest
by Dr. Ray Sahelian

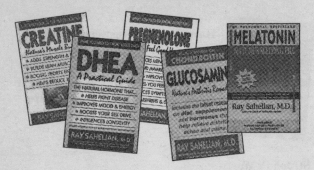

Creatine: Nature's Muscle Builder

Creatine, a combination of amino acids, has been found to be crucial for movement and muscle mass development. In this book, you will learn, in an easy-to-understand manner, how creatine works and what dosage is best for you. Paperback, 132 pages • $11.95 (Includes shipping & handling)

DHEA: A Practical Guide

This book discusses the safety of DHEA, how it affects the brain, heart, and immune system, and what is known about its anti-aging potential. More than 200,000 copies sold!
Paperback, 158 pages • $11.95 (Includes shipping & handling)

Pregnenolone: Nature's Feel Good Hormone

Find out how pregnenolone can improve vision, hearing, and mood. Pregnenolone can be used in hormone replacement therapy, and for conditions such as arthritis, depression, PMS, and various neurological disorders. Side effects are fully discussed.
Paperback, 157 pages • $11.95 (Includes shipping & handling)

Glucosamine: Nature's Arthritis Remedy

A full discussion of glucosamine hydrochloride and sulfate, and the role of chondroitin.
Paperback, 27 pages • $3.95 (Includes shipping & handling)

Melatonin: Nature's Sleeping Pill

Sleep like a baby, improve your mood, see vivid dreams, prevent jet lag, have more energy, and possibly live longer. The classic book on melatonin. Paperback, 157 pages • $11.95 (Includes shipping & handling)

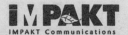

IMPAKT Communications

<u>BOOK YOUR PLACE ON OUR WEBSITE</u> AND MAKE THE <u>READING CONNECTION!</u>

We've created a customized website just for our very special readers, where you can get the inside scoop on everything that's going on with Zebra, Pinnacle and Kensington books.

When you come online, you'll have the exciting opportunity to:

- View covers of upcoming books
- Read sample chapters
- Learn about our future publishing schedule (listed by publication month *and author*)
- Find out when your favorite authors will be visiting a city near you
- Search for and order backlist books from our online catalog
- Check out author bios and background information
- Send e-mail to your favorite authors
- Meet the Kensington staff online
- Join us in weekly chats with authors, readers and other guests
- Get writing guidelines
- AND MUCH MORE!

**Visit our website at
http://www.kensingtonbooks.com**

EAT HEALTHY WITH KENSINGTON

COOKING WITHOUT RECIPES
by Cheryl Sindell   (1-57566-142-X, $13.00/$18.00)
Unleash your creativity and prepare meals your friends and family will
love with the help of this innovative kitchen companion. COOKING
WITHOUT RECIPES includes intriguing culinary strategies and nutritional secrets that will stir your imagination and put the fun back into
cooking.

EAT HEALTHY FOR $50 A WEEK
Feed Your Family Nutritious, Delicious Meals for Less
by Rhonda Barfield   (1-57566-018-0, $12.00/$15.00)
Filled with dozens of recipes, helpful hints, and sample shopping
lists, EAT HEALTHY FOR $50 A WEEK is an indispensable hand-
book for balancing your budget and stretching your groceries while
feeding your family healthy and nutritious meals.

THE ARTHRITIC'S COOKBOOK
by Collin H. Dong, M.D.   (1-57566-158-6, $9.95/$12.95)
and Jane Banks
Afflicted with debilitating, "incurable" arthritis, Dr. Collin H. Dong
decided to fight back. Combining traditional Chinese folk wisdom
with his western medical practice, he created a diet that made his
painful symptoms disappear. Today, used in conjunction with regular
arthritis medications, this groundbreaking diet has provided thousands
of Dr. Dong's patients with active, happy, and virtually pain-free lives.
It can do the same for you.